The Reality of Kriya Yoga

Inspiring Guidance From The Himalayan Master

Yogiraj Gurunath Siddhanath

2021

The Reality of Kriya Yoga
By Yogiraj Gurunath Siddhanath

First Edition Published in July 2021

Alight Publications
PO Box 277, Live Oak,
CA 95953

The Reality of KriyaYoga© 2021. All rights reserved by Sidhojirao Krishna Shitole. No part of this publication may be reproduced, stored in a retrieval system or database, or transmitted in any form or by any means electronic, mechanical, photocopying, recording, or otherwise without the prior written approval of the author or publisher.

ISBN 978-1-931833-55-4

Printed in the United States of America

THIS IS IT!
I HAVE REACHED HOME.
I HAVE QUENCHED
THE THIRST OF THE AGES

Forward

It is with excitement that we are able to take this opportunity to introduce you to the experiential words of a contemporary enlightened and God-Realized Master. He speaks to us in current cultural terms that we can relate with, rather than the antiquated terms from the old Masters of ancient times.

In the following pages are transcripts from Yogiraj's Satsangs where he answers the questions of spiritual seekers in his unique style. The unifying theme of this collection is the practical aspects of Kundalini Kriya Yoga that is offered by him for the purpose of guiding spiritual seekers onto the path of Self-Realization.

This is not a how-to-book and does not give instruction on techniques. Technques can be taught by teachers. What is more precious are the experiences that Yogiraj shares with us without holding back. He also give us what we need in the terms we can understand. He is not giving us theoretical information that is beyond our grasp.

During the process of editing, we were blessed with Yogiraj's personal attention. He spent several weeks of his precious time in correcting any mistakes and duplications as well as adding clarifications for the benefit of the reader.

I would like to thank all those who have contributed in one way or the other to the actualization of this book, from those who helped with the transcripts to those who helped to take the videos of Yogiraj's satsangs.

Jai Nath

Editor

Table of Contents

Part 1 Kriya Yoga

The Best Way to Dissolve Karma   /11
The Path of Yoga   /13
Kriya Yoga and Prana   /16
What does Kriya Yoga do to us when we practice?   /19
The Lightning Path   /20
What is Kriya Yoga   /23

Part II Master and Disciple

The Master dies to the disciple   /27
What is meant by idol worship as a sin?   /33
How the True Kriya Master overcomes ego   /35
Don't be a spoiled brat: Spiritual laws of patience and
    stress relief   /36
The Eternal Guru Principle revealed   /37
The Satguru helps you to get to God   /40
Kriya Yoga requires flexible disciple   /41
Awakening from Mindfulness to Soulfulness to Consciousness /44

Part III Discipline and Humility

Service and Devotion – Shakti and Bhakti   /47
Seva and Dissolving the Ego   /48
Individual Mind and Cosmic Consciousness   /55
The Prodigal son parable   /56
How to love and heal others as your larger self   /57
Physics nowhere now   /58
The so-called god particle   /59
Life is nothing more than this   /61
What is the source of your happiness?   /62
Self-Effort is the Key to Enlightenment   /62

Part IV Kriya and India Philosophy

Concentration, Meditation and the Power of Mind /67
Three Great Philosophies of India /68
God is the Supreme Reality /71
Is Kriya Yoga more advanced than Vipassana Meditation? /71
Origins of Tantra and Tantric Sex /73
Kundalini /77
Train the subconscious with Mantra /85
Intuition, Psychism and Ego: the limitations of
 interpreting Astrology /86
How can we accomplish anything while wanting
 to merge with nothing /90
Fate and Free Will /92

Part V Yogic Cosmology

Hold Steadfast to Practice /95
Yogic science of creation explained /95
 Psychological and Chronological Yugas of Time /97
The Rings pass not /99
Stages of samadhi and Shri Yukteswar's work in Hiranyaloka /101
The Cosmic Mind is Hiranya Garbha /107

Part VI Yoga and the West

Vegetarianism and Meditation /111
The Self – from Burning Man to Rainbow Man /112
The benefits of awakening Kundalini with the
science of Kriya Yoga /113
God is everywhere, so why meditate /114
Kriya and guilt fear complex /118
Invest in the everlasting /123

Part VII Experiences

Prepare for the experience of truth   /127
A Master Consciousness   /127
Meditate Share Care   /129
Allow Yourself to be Healed   /130
United Nations Experiential Address   /132
Be as a child of five   /137
Experiencing Divine Love   /138
Dreamweaver   /139
Ceremony - The Sacrament or Sacraments   /141
The Sacred Fire Ceremony   /142
Earth Peace Meditation   /145

Part VIII Miscellaneous Kriya Yoga Topics

The practice of Kriya Yoga – what you need to know   /149
What is Yoga?   /153
When Karma challenges Kriya practice, do this   /157
Kriya Yoga and the spine   /158
Kriya Yoga and Karma   /159
Interview Q&A   /161
Eliminate the I of the Ego to See the Eye or the Soul   /173
The Only Purpose of Our journey on This Earth
    is to Seek God   /174

Appendix

Yogiraj SatGurunath Siddhanath: A brief introduction   /179
Glossary   /183

More books by Yogiraj Gurunath Siddhanath   /205

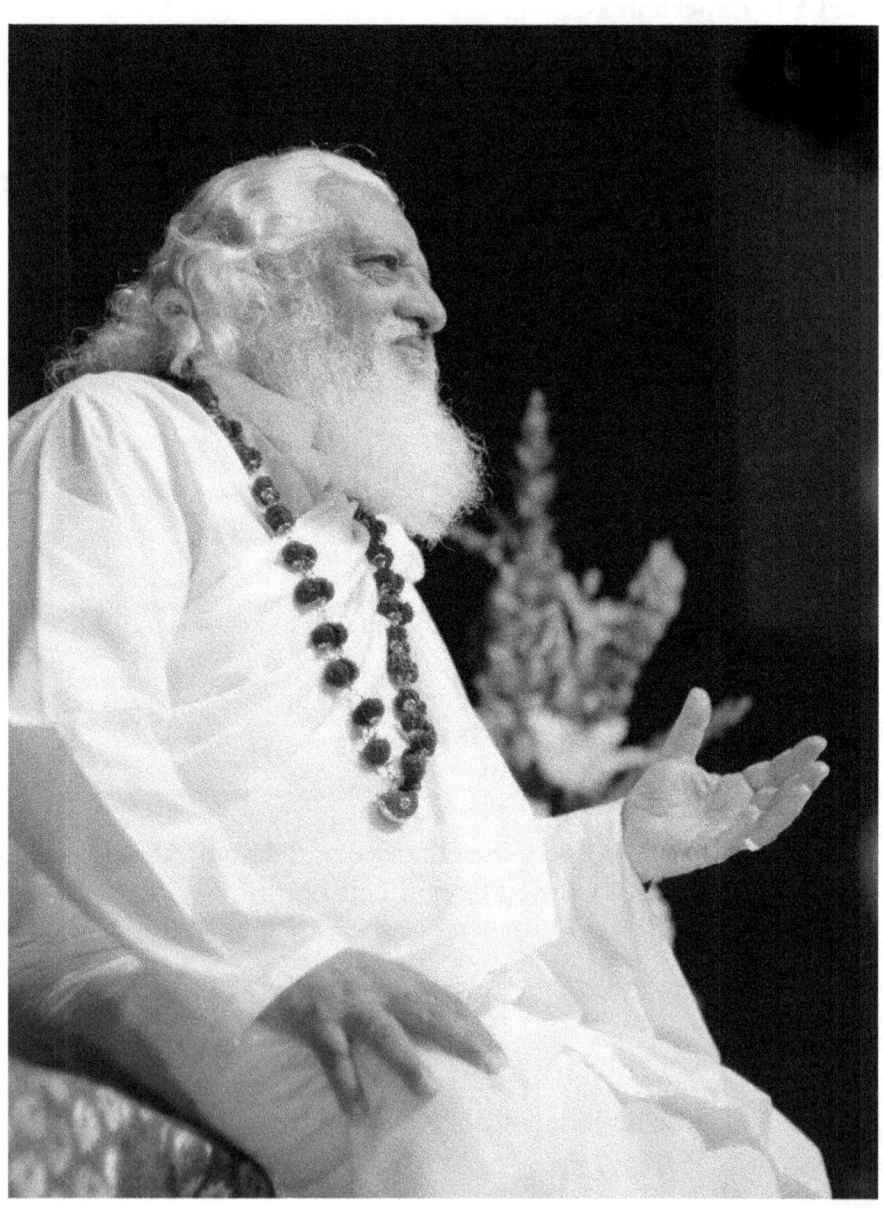

Part I
Kriya Yoga

REALITY OF KRIYA

Practice of the Kriya free
Is Soul's journey to Reality
One with your True Self to be

I practiced death with bated breath,
became breathless to death by breath
And Immortal have become!

But deathlessness to me
is naught unless
Divinity's Light shines forth!

Which melts even the immortal veil,
Maya's last effort to derail
My Soul's final journey to Reality

Not for the sake of deathlessness
but for the sake Divine
I transform immortality
by Awareness to Divinity!

Yogiraj Gurunath Siddhanath

The Best Way to Dissolve Karma

As the gentle abrasion of a river transforms a rough stone into a rounded Shivalinga. SO, the gentle abrasion of the Kriya breath transforms every Jiva into Shiva!

The Mahavatar Babaji Kriya Yoga is an Alchemy of Total Transformation. It is a dynamic process of Prana, breathing through the spinal cord, the spinal canal, and thereby transforming the latent impressions stored in your subconscious mind into positive life energy growth. When you move the breath of Kriya Yoga in your spinal cord, behind your vertebrae, there is a string, a tenuous, neuron-like thing, called the Sushumna Nadi, the spinal cord, within which is the Sushumna Nadi, Sushumna. When you move the breath in this channel, it is Kriya Yoga. This forms the bedrock and foundation of Raj Yoga into which Kriya transforms itself.

What does the breath do when it moves in the spine? It contacts certain astral plexes, known as the pranic lotuses, known as the chakras. And when it passes through the chakras, it nullifies your negative karma, along with bodily disease, mental disease of stress and tension, emotional suffering is all transformed to positive life energy growth, which finally evolves you to a contentless Consciousness. Each individual has his own set of genomes, his DNA. In the DNA – DNA stands for Dioxyribonucleic Acid – so say the scientists. But that is only a shadow of the pranic chakras, which are the true source, the vortex of energy, which link the spiritual to the material. So, when these chakras have generated a house, made a house for themselves called the DNA. Now, the DNA has on it what is called nitrogen nubs, four nitrogen nubs. They are like tape recorders. And they fill, it's like a DVD. Like in Europe, they say DVD [German pronunciation]. So, it's a DVD, which records all your past deeds and actions. Nobody can escape from it, you know? If you say I'm a great dietitian and going in the night to your fridge and eating the best of chocolates, it's all recorded in the DNA, the DVD. And it's not only in audio cassette. The damn problem is that it's a DVD!

So, if I sit like this and from my projector, I project my DVD, then you can see on the screen my whole life story of past, present and future. Now, the Kriya breath. That's the great, divine genius of Babaji. What does the Kriya breath do? Kriya breath, while moving through the spinal cord. And Gurunath, how do we make the breath move through the spinal cord? By intent. There's a saying in Yogic Parlance. Wherever the concentrated mind is, there the Prana shall be. So as you move your Prana, concentrating in the narrow pathway, the Pilgrim's Progress, in the spinal cord, this breath, this pranic life energy, rubs out the tape on the DNA. The tape recorder can be rubbed out and nullified. That's why this is a dynamic process, and a very scientific process.

That's why the oldest tradition in the world is the tradition of the Siddhas. They straddle Buddhism, they straddle Jainism, they straddle the Yogis of the Garhwal Himalayas. And older than the Siddha tradition are the elite of the Siddhas, who are ever immortal, they are called the Nath Yogis. Nath Siddhas. The Siddhanaths. Now this oldest of tradition, wanted to expound, this technique, this dynamic process of evolution, the evolution of spiritual consciousness to the west. Therefore, they had to take somebody, somebody, put in it some soul of a Yogi, they put in this body my soul, given me this body.

It's okay. I've got a broken leg and a cracked-up skull, not much brains. But they made a useful guy out of this body. And he has to relate and translate to them in this digital, scientific language, before he goes to the devotional language.

So, when this breath moves in the DNA, it has an abrasive action on the DNA, that is the life energy and the DNA create a motion. This abrasion transforms Karma – how many of you know, or have heard of the word Karma, raise your hand. But now I'm going to tell you how the Karma, where it is lodged and how it can be transformed, which none of the techniques here tell you. For sixty years plus, I've done Yoga and nothing Yoga, and I've been to all the systems and everywhere, and that's where the genius of Babaji lies in the fact, that this is the only technique that can transform your negative Karma. It transforms negative Karmas and simultaneously evolves your consciousness.

This is what the Kriya Yoga does. It's very important to understand this. That it's a dynamic process of the evolution of spiritual consciousness. It is very simple – the more absorption, the more concentration you do it with, the more you will be absorbed. That means the more concentration you will do it, the more you will slip into meditation and Samadhi. I hear people say here, "I'm going to meditate. I'm going to do this; I'm going to do that." You cannot meditate! "I'm going to open the flower. This is a beautiful bud of a sunflower, of a lotus or a rose, I'm going to open it." No, no. You have to water the plant, and the flower will open itself, otherwise you'll break the petals. Aye?

Samadhi happens as a result of Meditation. Meditation happens as a result of concentration. Concentration is the practice of spiritual growth. You must know it.

This happens as a result of Pratyahara which happens as a result of Kriya Pranayama. Yoga is all connected in a sequence. The Kriya Pranayama is the foundation and the pinnacle. It transform jiva soul to Spirit Atma.

The Path of Yoga

The purpose of Yoga is to merge into divine consciousness. And in this instance, Kriya Yoga in particular, we could say is to comprehend God in a final state called Kavalya (the enlightened awareness of total satisfaction). So how do we comprehend that Reality which is beyond mind by a limited mind? What seems like an impossible dichotomy to the mind, which to the Yogis is very achievable through the tried and tested practice of Yoga. In Yoga the first physical stage of this comprehension, begins from preparing the body to be healthy, to be fit, have no aches and pains, have a healthy digestive and circulatory system by the practice of Yoga Asanas, they create a healthy body mind system.

> As a leaking vessel never can fill,
> The waters of life so pure and still
> So distracted mind fails to retain
> Wisdom's nectar in its brain.

For the practicing yogi a concentrated mind is of prime importance, and the process of circulation, assimilation and elimination is also the power of God working in the body. In the next level of comprehending God through Yoga, the practitioner finds that the balsam of yogic breath soothes turbulent emotions – the hurt and the suffering – refining and transforming them to devotion and love. All the insults that the person has borne, all the hardships, the treacheries that the near and dear ones have committed, all these traumatic scars are healed by the rhythmic devotional breath of Kundalini Pranayama. In the mental process, the same pranayama – the practice of systematic rhythmic breathing – cures psychosomatic disorders, like ulcers and asthma and sclerosis, by calming the mind.

> To ease disease of random mind
> A remedy suitable we must find
> A rhythmic breathing tension free
> With Kriya Yoga the sovereign key.

The moving to the next stage, the emotions that are hurt are transformed into devotion and life, becoming a flowing stream towards God in pratyahara, which gives rise to Love. This manifests in devotional chanting, singing Christmas carols, singing God's praise, bhajans and hymns. The process of refining carries on step by step through consistent Yoga practice. Then as the yogi begins to concentrate (dharana) and meditate (dhyan), the mind gradually becomes a placid crystal pool. The undisturbed crystal mind is a beautiful mind.

> Steady poise the arrow of your will
> And shoot the fleeting mind to still
> The deer of thoughts hinds and harts
> Felled by your concentrated darts.

Then begins the journey through various states of samadhi. This thought-free state becomes the constant state of the yogi's mind. With additional practice of special techniques given by the Satguru, the mind is gradually transcended, leading to an internal glow.

> As one by one they die away
> Mind opens up to new day
> Where streams run tranquil and willows sway
> Here tame and gentle deer do play.

Mind you, the practitioner has still not yet reached the state of comprehending an incomprehensible God, but step-by-step through the practice of Yoga, the yogi is getting there. Continuing the journey of Yoga, the yogi gets into states of mysticism. From and unkempt, disheveled and disorderly mind, the yogi has organized the mind, and the mind dissolves into the opal glow of divinity. Becoming one with it, the yogi gradually transforms to light. The refinement of the mind continues further, and the consciousness expands and intuition sharpens. The yogis get visions of gods and saints and goddesses. A vision of the beautiful Krishna, of Christ. Walking with Jesus, transported way back three thousand years, walking along the sea of Galilee, the yogi may or may not realize himself or herself to be a disciple – Simon, Peter or Paul – or connected to other masters from before. From this state of Savikalpa Samadhi, the constantly striving yogi is ready to move into more profound states. After getting these deep intuitions and finishing with them, the yogi gets to the Mount of Olives, contacting the higher portion of Jesus, the son of man, and Christ, the Son of God. The Christ state of temporary Nirvikalpa Samadhi is a radiant aura of Opal glow. The yogi merges into that aura, and here there's no form or figure, just an eternal bliss called the Christ Consciousness – Krishna Consciousness.

> Then tamed and tuned to nature's flow,
> Mind melts into an opal glow
> Which radiates from the soul within
> Where wisdom's mystic fire is king.

This is what the persistent gradual practice of Yoga does; from curing a practitioner's pain and headaches to getting into the state of Nirvikalpa Samadhi. And in the transfiguration, the trinity in creation-Brahma, Vishnu, Mahesh- but is transformed into their formless attributes. Finally moving further from the Christ state, the Yogi gets into the ineffable state of the Christos, Shiva-Goraksha-Babaji, the Babaji state of comprehending the Reality. But this, my dear souls, is not the final stage yet because the Yogi not only has to comprehend the God who is incomprehensible but also the God who is complete and therefore also comprehensible, complete, and incomplete. All dualities have to transform and merge for the Yogi to achieve this state. The Isness of the zero-not-zero. The Yogi then in this ultimate leap merges into the finality of the comprehensible and the not comprehensible, the zero and the not zero, whose center is everywhere and circumference nowhere, the state of Niranjan Nirvan, Kaivalya. I address this Consciousness simply as the Isness. That's where the finality of Yoga takes one, to the true innermost being who is one with the Supreme Being. The only One I know who came back from the State of No Return is Shiva-Goraksha-

Babaji.

Kriya Yoga and Prana

So, I have a number of questions for you, and the first one that I want to ask is, as a living Kriya Yoga master, how would you describe Kriya Yoga to the layperson?

Kriya Yoga is a simple science of life energy control. I would describe it as a pranic meditation – a meditation done with pranayama. There are two currents in the body – prana and apana. The pranic current flows from the base of the spine up to the third eye. It's a unifying and evolving current. It evolves consciousness. The apanic current flows from the third eye down the spine to the base – to the root chakra. This apanic current burns all negativity and past evil karma. At the physical level, you can say it is a rejuven-detox technique. The upward-flowing current of prana rejuvenates the body cells and the downward current of apana destroys all negativity and toxins in the body. So, a rejuven-detox technique at the physical level. At the spiritual level, the upward breath of prana evolves consciousness and the downward apanic current burns your past evil karma. This is a simple way of describing Kriya Yoga, and I always tell my disciples one thing: that just as the gentle abrasion of a river transforms all the stones into the form of a Shivalinga – it rounds them off, so also the gentle abrasion of Kriya Yoga wears away the rough edges of the personality and makes of every jiva a Shiva. So the practice of the gentle abrasion of the breath, the constant moving of the breath, transforms jiva into Shiva. This is the efficacy and importance of Kriya Yoga. It is simple; anyone can do it, and it is meant for everyone.

Simply put, how would you describe prana for the layperson?

Prana is an internal energy of the body. In English, for lack of a better word, they call it life force. In all these movies and all, you see "may the force be with you" and all that, but when they say "may the force be with you", they're very new to the version of pranayama, so they call it force. It's a force – a dynamic energy. That's what prana is associated with, and they say that prana permeates the whole universe. From the smallest atom to the vastest galaxy, it is animated by prana – the exhalation of creation. The exhalation of the Creator. And the inhalation gives life – prana vivifies nature. Prana puts life into inert matter, and therefore prana is the basic substratum of the livingness of creation. That's how I would describe prana.

And what is contained in prana that makes it such a force for evolution – the essential element of evolution? What is that?

The outermost form of prana is the breath, which we can compare to the electric wire. Then prana itself we can compare to the electricity which runs in the electric wire. So, just as the electricity runs in the electric wire, so also prana runs through the breath to give us life. Behind prana is the light of livingness which we associate with the direct Shakti – the direct divinity of God; the dynamic kundalini energy of God. So behind the prana is that living-ness of light. Prana is half terrestrial; the middle portion of prana is celestial, and the source of prana is divine. So prana is a bridge between humanity, the celestial regions, and divinity. Therefore, prana is very important in the evolution of the human being as a whole and human consciousness specifically.

What you're saying is, is that there is a consciousness that is infused in the breath that we take, that is at the same time celestial and divine, and that is the thing that gives us life? Like a cosmic intelligence carried in the breath – would that be a way to say it?

Yes. The cosmic intelligence is infused into the force – the life energy – of prana. Prana itself lends motion to the breath, and breath itself moves in the body through its lungs to animate the body for its living activities. Therefore, when we take medicines or tonics, the medicines are not healing you. It is the prana, which is the master mason that builds your body cells, which is the body doctor. The master mason and body doctor of healing is prana, and not the medicines. The prana works through the medicines – the medicines are a catalyst. They make prana available. They invoke prana and prana heals your body.

Prana evolves your consciousness because consciousness can relate directly with prana and celestial energy rather than directly with matter. Prana is the bridge between humanity and Divinity.

We're breathing all day long – without breath, we die – so what is it that makes the breath and the divine or celestial intelligence in the breath work to evolve or to heal a person as opposed to just a regular keep-me-alive kind of breath? What's the difference

So, the difference is your awareness of the willingly intent to Pranic breath that, when you're breathing normally, prana is moving your breath normally, but when you want to direct prana for a specific purpose, it is intent that matters. The faculty of exclusive attention, if you apply it to the breath moving, the concentration will draw the prana to that particular spot or place which needs to be healed. The degree of concentration applied will be your success in pranayama, whether it be for self-evolution or healing. . The degree of focused attention is important to achieve the results. But after a certain stage, when you are so focused, the attention snaps and you're floating in that focused-ness. When you are focusing effortlessly, that dharana, or concentration, becomes dhyana. And when you go into a deeper state of dharana where your effortless focus makes you forget yourself and you become the object your are focusing on, that is called Savikalpa Samadhi. And when there is no object to focus on and you're focusing on the divine awareness with nothing as its object and you've lost body consciousness, that is called Nirvikalpa Samadhi – samadhi without any vikalpa. These are the states of Samadhi.

So, the important thing to develop as a faculty in our practice is the ability to not doubt – to be super-clear about what's possible when we put our mind to this because the breath will do the rest. So it's what I call taming the mind-monkeys – the things that keep us jumping around in the mind. That's really what it comes down to at the most basic level, and then to become what I've heard you call no-mind, that's a much further evolution.

Yes. These are preliminary things. Firstly, a person who doubts and disbelieves will not come to practice yoga. He won't come to an ashram, because he'll be having his own ideology, whatever it is – car racing or gambling or just going for exercise. But the people who are focused on this already have that confidence and already know the import of yoga. They know the import of yoga and the value of yoga, and they have no doubt that it evolves them from man the brute to man the man to man the god or woman the brute to woman the woman to woman the goddess.

Now, talking about the mind-which has all monkey thoughts. . I give the mind monkey work by Kriya Yoga. The mind is the monkey of thoughts, so I make him go down with the down-going breath and I make the monkey go up with the up-coming breath till all the distracting thoughts fade away. So, give the monkey some work by climbing up and down the pole. We tire the mind by going up and down and up and down until the mind gets more and more refined and purifies to a state of Divine mind and no distracting thoughts come – only the Chaitanya prana is moving up and down the central column.

What Does Kriya Yoga Do To Us When We Practice?

Now let us get to the simple science of Kriya Yoga – Kundalini Kriya Yoga. When we practice Kundalini Kriya Yoga, we use two main pranic currents of the body to get into a state of dharana, dhyana, and samadhi, and those currents are prana and apana.

So what is the pranic current and what is the apanic current? The pranic current rises up the spinal cord from the muladhara chakra. It rises up the spinal canal. It is soothing and calm and evolving in nature – it evolves human consciousness. So this pranic current rises up the spine from the muladhara chakra to the agya chakra. It is satwik; it is expanding in nature and leads to dhyan, dharana, and samadhi. The second current which we breathe is known as the apanic current, which starts from the third eye – kutastha chaitanya – and it goes downwards, burning all negativity.

The true practice of Kundalini Kriya Yoga is prana-apana yagna – you offer the fire of prana and apana. As Lord Sri Krishna says in the Gita, when we breathe and do the prana-apana fire ceremony – the prana-apana yagna – the disease, decay and death of our body is eliminated as we practice the Kundalini Kriya Yoga. The down-going breath of apana destroys all negativity and negative karma and the upcoming breath of prana evolves human consciousness. The effect of Kriya is like a double-edged sword, the Excalibur.

An encouraging message

So, this is very, very important to know, dear souls – that the only purpose of your sojourn on Earth is to seek God. All other things are important but are secondary to atma-vidya. The experiential satsang, of course, is to give you the confidence and the faith that you will not be wasting your time by practising the science of selfing into the self, but you will be evolving from moment to moment. With every breath, you will be creating God within you. What a wonderful thought – what a wonderful idea. Keep the highest goal. Merge your soul into the spirit of the universal divine consciousness.

Babaji Kriya Yoga Secrets – The Lightning Path

Now when you do this sadhana – shwasa dhane sadhana – the breath is the practice of spiritual growth. When you constantly breathe, it gets subtler and subtler into life-energy and when you get life-energy control, it dissolves the Karma which is latent in the pranic lotuses of your spine. So, your destiny is in your spine, your destiny is in your spine. So, therefore, it does give you something to strive for – because the only purpose of man's sojourn on this earth is to seek God. But the question is – It is so slow. If I'm chanting, "Om Namah Shivay, Hare Ram, Hare Krishna, Krishna Krishna, Hare Hare, Hare Ram Hare," I will get there, no doubt, I will get there. Even if I start walking from here to Santa Clara, definitely I'll get there. But if I take a car, I will get there faster. So, this is the lightning path.

God is behind every good action

People of eagle hearts cannot wait to see their beloved. But their beloved is God, camouflaged behind the smile of a loving girlfriend, camouflaged in the beautiful red Ferrari. And they are very possessive. It's good here in America, I saw a guy with a Ferrari and at the back number plate it was written: She's red, she's hot and she's mine. You want to totally possess that car. So, I asked him where's your girlfriend, he said, it doesn't matter it's this thing. You touch his car, he says, "don't touch the car!" So that's his new girlfriend. That's okay! But it is God which is giving him the joy behind the Ferrari. It's God which is giving you the joy behind the loving arms of your husband. It's God that is behind, giving you the joy of the food that your wife cooks for you. Everything behind every good action is God, but you get deluded into these minor things and forget the goal. All these are evanescent joys – a flash in the pan – the Everlasting

Joy is God alone.

They tried – Leonard Orr tried to bring a technique of Haidakhan Babaji. I had a talk with Haidakhan Babaji I told him this is Leonard Orr, and he's going off the track. Instead of teaching preaching divinity, he preached immortality. Immortality is a by-product of divinity, not immortality for itself. Also, the Nath yogis and the siddhas of the Himalayas do not do body immortality for the sake of immortality. They keep a fine body – the rainbow body full of light – free from the ravages of time – not because they want a divine body of rainbow light free from ravages of time, because but because they want such a body so that in a healthy body temple, they can house a healthy God and more of the divinity will come into them. So, divinity, God, the divine consciousness itself is the sole purpose of your sojourn on this earth, not the yogic beauty spa of body immortality. That's the spa. And if you go to the yogic spa your cells will stop degenerating. They will stop. But that will happen – don't focus on that. That will happen by virtue of your yearning for God. It takes a long time! If I go from L.A. to Santa Clara walking or to San Francisco it will take me some days. If I go by car it's faster. If I go by the speed of light, it'll take me eight minutes from here to sun, or take me a few seconds from here to the moon. It's faster. But if I have to cross the universe – if I have to cross the universe at the speed of light – then it will take ten billion light years. But if I travel at seventy billion times the speed of light it will take me two-and-a-half to three months to cross the whole universe.

So this is the expanse, but what happens in meditation? Light, space, and time become gravitational. It becomes the guruthva – the gravity of the inner knowing of God and God has no time, He has centres everywhere, his circumferences nowhere. He is boundless. That is the person about whom we are talking, about whom we are searching. Of course, I cannot tell you the essence of it; I can only tell the pointers. I can tell you about you – how you can get to the Being about whom naught may be said. So I am talking about everything but that Being about whom naught may be said. But still it is so encouraging, it points the direction, it gives you the way, it shows you the light. What does the Guru do? He is the lighthouse. He is the navigator. He shows you the light, avoiding the pitfalls which he has been through, but which you don't have to go through. Therefore, it's necessary for a Master to guide the disciple along the path.

Now it takes a million million years to express cosmic consciousness, which is also called the Krishna consciousness. This is all self-realisation, just a wee-bit below God-realisation. It's also called the Christ consciousness. It is called the Nath Mandal – that's connected with us – the Nath Mandal or the Buddha field. So, to get to the Buddha field, to get to your beloved Krishna or your Christ or your Divine Goddess, whoever, you would not like to practice for a million, million years. It's too long for the brain cells to express cosmic consciousness.

Kriya Yoga – Babaji's Kriya Yoga is the lightning path. It is the lightning path which makes you speed up your evolution. And I'm giving you approximation. If you do 144 of the Kriya you will reach in a certain time. If you, do it faster, if you do ten to sixteen hours, eighteen hours a day, you will get self-realized in three years. If you do eight to ten hours a day, it will take you six years. If you do about six to eight hours a day, it will take you about twelve years. And if you do two hours to three hours a day, it will take you 24 years. So, two to three hours or two hours is enough. That is the group which I'm dealing with here – about one to two hours a day, which they can comfortably do without upsetting their day-to-day programme, their chores. So, they've got a lot of time to run their errands. But then who's going to run the errand of God? We have God's errands to run also. And where do we run God's errands? We run them in the spinal cord. Up and down and up and down till the messenger of the errand, the errand itself, and God become one. This is the purpose of running all errands – to become one with the errand and the object. So, this is what Kriya Yoga is all about. It is called the lightning path also. It speeds up the evolution of consciousness.

I'm not here to teach you any religion or cult. I'm not here to convert you to Islam, neither am I here to make you a Jehovah's Witness or a Hare Krishna or a Shaivite or a siddha yogi. I'm here to tell you about you. I'm here to tell you about you. And therefore, I tell you that the community that we form, we must all realise that: "Humanity is our uniting religion, Breath our uniting prayer (which we will be doing in Kriya Yoga) and Consciousness our uniting God." Those who don't want to breathe need not breathe with us. Those who don't accept themselves as human beings need not join our community humanity. So, 'community humanity' is very small at the moment, in this frame of definition, but in truth, it is the whole of the human race. We have a following, we have a group of like-minded people, of fact-minded people, of over seven billion people. That's our database! That's the population of the people on Earth.

Anything less that this would create a cult. Christianity, Buddhism, Hinduism, Islam are all cults. But Humanity is not cult. Humanity is the existence of souls on this earth who want to realize the true nature of their Being.

The initiation into the Babaji's Kriya Yoga, every time you get it, helps your life-energy to flow and assists in the expansion of your consciousness. The practice of one half a minute cycle of Kriya Yoga is equal to one year of natural spiritual progress. Evolution to become one with the Reality can be expedited tremendously by going in higher and higher states of Samadhi.

What is Kriya Yoga?

I am speaking to you about the science of Kriya Yoga which has its process rooted in the soil of love. Kriya Yoga is a very simple process of spinal breathing. Anyone can do it and everyone can do it. It is for you. It is the gift from Shiva-Goraksha-Babaji to the present humanity to override all crisis situations, to override all the difficulties which come along the path as you live your life. Nobody has it easy these days, everyone is struggling, and everybody is going through difficult times. Some are going through good times. But whatever the situation, the practice of Kriya Yoga, the evolution of human consciousness, will stand you in good stead. Kriya Yoga is a state of awareness – dynamic awareness.

Kri means to do, and Yoga means to unite. By the spiritual doing, by the spiritual practice, you may unite to the divine in-dweller which lies at the core of your own being. "Yoga is an inner ascent through ever more refined and ever more expanded spheres of mind to get to the divine consciousness, to get to the God Essence which lies at the core of your own being." So, it's an inner ascent. Yoga is nothing less than the union of your individual soul with universal spirit. It has nothing to do directly with Hatha, or what you call the practice of the physical postures, or the breathing or the pranayam. They are all essential in the sense that they are assisting and composing the main practice of Yoga. Kriya Yoga begins with the Pranic Meditation of Raj Yoga, it takes you right up to Samadhi. The main practice of Yoga, and what Yoga consists of, is divided into eight portions, which unite as one. This is called Ashtanga Yoga. Yama, niyama, asana, pranayama, pratyahara, dharana, dhyana and samadhi. These are the eight limbs of Yoga. They collectively may be called Yoga: That is the Union with the Divine. But any one of them alone cannot be called Yoga. If you want to call any one single thing Yoga, then it is samadhi: "Yogaha samadhi." And samadhi means the highest state even after Zen, Satori or the lower state of rejuvenation. samadhi means consciousness of expanded ecstasy. So, when your consciousness expands into the thought free state of knowing bliss that is the state of samadhi. That is the state of enlightenment. And this is what Kriya Yoga gets you to. Out of compassion for humanity lost in delusion and error, Goraksha Babaji gave the Householders Kriya Yoga. Kriya Yoga is householders' yoga in today's world. In the practical application of a person's day-to-day life: their earnings, their jobs, their peace of mind and inner calm. At the physical level I call it the Rejuven-Detox technique.

Kriya is not a cult or creed or religion. Kriya Yoga is a way of life which helps you to do what you are already doing better. If you are a Protestant Christian, it will make you better Protestant. If you are a Catholic, a better Catholic. So, in uniting the world Kriya Yoga has a very vital role to play. Kriya Yoga is a simple practice of spinal breathing – an upward breath and a downward breath – connected with two body currents called prana and apana. Pranic current flows from the base of the spine to the third eye. It calms the mind and soothes the nerves. It takes you into state of expanded awareness. And the other current you have to deal with is apanic current, which is flowing from the third eye to the root chakra. So, the pranic current is Shiva and the apanic current is Shakti. The pranic current which moves up evolves consciousness. The apanic current which moves down the spine dissolves and burns all your negative Karma. As you practice, these two breaths even themselves out and you are in the still breath state after many months or years or lifetimes and know your mind to be crystal and quiet. Know your mind to be in state of perfect tranquillity or composed mind. This is Samadhi.

Yogiraj Gurunath Siddhanath

Part II
Master and Disciple

*From my own Being I have
woven the web of my ashram
And those who get caught in
the net of my freedom shall
never be in bondage again.*

Nath gives the desireless state of total satisfaction

The Reality of Kriya Yoga

The Master Dies to the Disciple

The master's outer form dies to the disciple to the extent of the degree of his concentration on the master. Let's say this is the master here – a person called Yogiraj Gurunath. For all practical purposes, this is the master and there's the disciple. The disciple is focusing on the master. The master is sitting before you, in one place, and he is also part of the inner most essence of your true self. He's in two places, in your heart and here. He is subjectively in your heart and objectively here. Is that clear? Now you begin to concentrate on the master. As you concentrate, you will find your thoughts are running away, but then you bring it back to his face, his hair, his beard, and you are beginning to say, "oh, beloved Master, I am so happy to have you because when I see your face, I forget all my outward distractions. I forget all my going shopping, even though it's Christmas time and you look like Santa Claus."

I mean, I'm just giving you a sample prayer. Whatever prayer you know, keep praying. As you keep praying, the Master creates a magnetism on his face and in your heart and you get connected to his face. This is a dynamic process of factual Samadhi which I am taking you through. It's a dynamic progression. It's an actual happening – experiential Samadhi.

And the atoms of the disciple's eyes and the master's atoms get connected into one form. And the gaze of the disciple steadies on the Master. His mind stops running. The Master is called Guru. The word "Guru" comes from "Gurutva" and "Gurutvakarshan," which is magnetic or gravitational attraction. So as the Master does his gravitational effect, Gurutva means gravity. The Guru is one who has the gravity to bring out the hidden knowledge of the disciple and enlighten him. This is my description. He cracks the code of Maya and takes you to the Reality. That is the SatGuru.

So, as you continue, the Guru starts dissolving – his form starts dying into the concentration of the disciple, which now turns into a meditation. Then there's no distraction of thought. The disciple keeps looking at the Master and Satguru. The Satguru helps the disciple in a uniform, double way, by creating an attraction in the heart of the disciple. That is one of the places where he is. The disciple keeps looking with interest at the Guru's face and steadies his mind. The leaking wounds of distracted thoughts have disappeared, and the mind is solid and now in a state of meditation. His thoughts are not wavering anywhere, and the Guru is gradually dying into the disciple by his gravity and merging into the disciple. The disciple's atoms are one with the atoms of the Guru and he has become an integral part of the disciple's meditation. From concentration, the disciple has gone to a deeper layer of meditation. Formerly, in concentration, the Guru was an integral part of him, but now he and the Guru are one. The whole of the Guru and the disciple have become one in meditation. As the disciple keeps looking at the SatGuru, who further moves into the disciple's awareness and makes the disciple enter from the atomic to the sub-atomic layer. The Guru loses form. The eyes of the disciple are fixed on the Guru and the disciple can see the aura around the Guru. The aura is expanding more and more. It's a white cottony gold with flashes of violet, purple, rose and indigo – rose-coloured and golden coloured. And the disciple keeps looking, his eyes are watering not blinking.

The SatGuru's form is disappearing. He goes to the formless state. That means the disciple and the Master have entered from the atomic structure to the sub-atomic structure of the Guru's form where they see not his form so clearly, but they feel the joy. They see his attributes. So you do not see the Guru's face or his beard so clearly, but are now beginning to experience his sub-atomic energy of ananda. So this is the third stage. The SatGuru has died from the form and become a formless ananda in the heart of the disciple. This is how the Guru gradually dissolves himself and dies to the disciple, killing the ego of the disciple in the process.

In the next stage, the disciple now experiences only the energy of the SatGuru. From an integral part, the disciple becomes the whole of the Guru. From a part of his energy of joy of ananda, now the disciple concentrates deeper and goes into an ecstasy of expanded consciousness where he realises himself and the joy of the Guru in all completeness. First, he realised the attribute of joy partially, but now he goes deeper to realise it completely. And at this stage, which is the state of Savikalpa Savikalpa samadhi, 'crack-patack', the ego has split. He has cracked the code. His ego has dissolved. And he is now floating in a vast sea of satchidananda.

Then as he goes deeper, the master dissolves himself into the disciple in the final stage. Where he appears to the disciple and the disciple experiences himself as a vast undifferentiated consciousness of radiant ether – a homogeneous energy of radiant ether. And his mind is expanded to the far limits of the mind and matter of the universe. He is everywhere. His mind has become crystal thought of existence, consciousness and bliss. He is existence, consciousness, and bliss. He has no thought, just the feeling of deep peace and subtle waves of joy. He has no desire, neither for himself, nor for his Guru, nor for God, knowing that he's experiencing God and floating in a vast sea of joy. So, the Master has died for the disciple to become a sea of joy. He's cracked his ego and disappeared and become the experience of disciple's samadhi.

Now he's in a state of self-realization and the disciple's mind is called the bearer of truth because he can see the universal energies working in tandem, working in karma. His mind has expanded to the size of the universe. He has realized God, but only through Divine Mind. Now in the crucial state. He must take the quantum leap – the paradigm shift from Divine Mind to Divine Consciousness – and nobody can do it for him. If he tries, he fails, because in this state of mind, there is no desire, and to try means he has a desire. If the disciple doesn't try, he's also stuck, because no effort is made to penetrate the star of mind. He just has to wait in innocent awareness in all humility for the grace of God. In that state, God the Guru will come.

The whole energy of the universe is like a whole ocean of molten glass. It's a homogeneous fabric of radiant ether, without a ripple of thought. This will coalesce into a huge star, and the disciple will be pulled through his own star gate by the gravity of Gurukrupa. That is the grace of the Guru. No ego, no I, no effort, no practice of Kriya Yoga, nothing will do it. You just have to be. Then stiller than stillness itself with bated breath I do behold, thy rising self star's nectar gold. And then by Gurutvakarshan, he's pulled through the gate of his own Divine Mind. And he enters from a state of self-realization to a state of God Realization. He enters from a state of Savikalpa Samadhi to Nirvikalpa Samadhi. He enters from the spheres of relativity into the state beyond relativity. He has passed the rings past not, by constantly being in this state, practising the state of Savikalpa Samadhi. This is the manner in which the Guru dies unto the disciple and he leads him from one stage to a higher, subtler stage of consciousness. And when the disciple has passed from a state of self-realization of Divine Mind, he takes the form of a huge star. The disciple passes through his own star gate, falls into eternity, and falls into his own gravity – his own Gurutvakarshan. Gurutvakarshan, spiritual gravity, goes in through the star gate. You've all heard of star gate. It's within you. He passes through the star gate. He goes into eternity, or she goes into eternity. Then they go into a state of Divine Consciousness. But here as the valiant yogi constantly practices, Asamprajnata Samadhi or Nirvikalpa Samadhi, again and again, he's conquered his thoughts. He's conquered his thought forms. His thoughts are Vritti, he's conquered Chitta Vritti Nirodha . He's conquered his Chitta Vritti, his thoughts, his worldly thoughts. He's conquered his thought forms, which are Pratyahara. But he's not conquered, even in a state of Divine Mind, he has not permanently conquered what is called his 'remembered experiences of past lives,' which is Samskar. He's a totally enlightened being, but he's not liberated. He's not got to Brahma Nirvana and he's not got to Nirvana Moksha.

There lies the difference between enlightenment and the permanent state of Brahma Nirvana.

We use the word enlightenment loosely. There are many stages of enlightenment. As the disciple practices, flying from Divine Mind of self-realization to Divine Consciousness of God Realization, again and again he's pulled back to Divine Mind because desires of past lives bubble on the surface of his mind's lake, to pull the Hamsa – the soul swan – back again to relativity. Then again, the valiant yogi tries again for Nirbeeja Samadhi. You see, unless the samadhi is less than one seed of thought, of all your past, present and future lives, you cannot be liberated. You cannot get nirvana moksha. You can only be enlightened into that state – if you got that state, you know it in Divine Mind. And as he practices, year after year, decade after decade, life after life, the desires of past lives, stored impressions of past lives, remembered experiences, bubble up from the surface of his mind's lake to pull the soul swan back into the lake of Divine Mind. And again the valiant soul makes his effort, and rises above the lake of Divine Mind to enter Nirvikalpa Samadhi, Asamprajnata samadhi, the state of Divine Consciousness. And then again, a thousand years ago, he had had a love affair with some name, and that thought pulls him back. Again, he must trace it, suppress it, and transform it, and again take the flight. A million times this will happen. And a million time the valiant soul will fly. He will make his effort or he will just stay in the state of passive alertness. So, you cannot try and you cannot not try. To get from a state of Savikalpa Samadhi to Nirvikalpa Samadhi, from Self

Realization to God Realization, you cannot try and you cannot not try. You just have to be. You have to be in a state of innocent, passive awareness. No bhakti, no shakti, just be. God knows it all. You're already connected. You have to let that boil down. You have to let the heat subside. You have to let the thought and desire finish. Even the last thought of desire, unless it is finished, you cannot get to the permanent. And then after long, long lifetimes, you, the soul swan, shall win your wings to freedom. You and your master, your Satguru, will be one. Such is the work of the Satguru. He takes you from self-realization to Divine Realization.

Once you have Divine Realization, there is no Kriya Yoga. There is no Kriya movement. Kriya is right up to the state of Savikalpa Samadhi. And the effort of sitting again, to Nirvikalpa Samadhi. But then when you're in a permanent state of Nirvikalpa Samadhi – of no thought, no mind – when you're permanently at that state, there's no desire at all – of person, place or thing, or of present, past or future lives. And your mind is totally crystal. Nay, not totally crystal – the mind itself is totally dissolved. As the whole universe, as from the first, was a state of undifferentiated, radiant ether, your mind was a fabric of an undifferentiated, radiant ether. Now your mind has become a fabric of undifferentiated, radiant light. First it was undifferentiated, radiant electron, but remember that the electron is one mile slower than light.

Then in Nirvikalpa Samadhi, you become the undifferentiated, radiant light, so you and your Guru are one. The Guru has died unto you. He has died unto your ego, to kill your ego and liberate you from the trammels of the senses. And he has taken you from your mind and state to the whole sum and substance of the far limits of the universe. The far energy that reaches the universe of mind and matter. The far limits of mind and matter. From the fabric of undifferentiated, radiant electron, one electron, that electron becomes fluid and flows into the fabric in Nirbeeja Samadhi, in God consciousness. Just before you get to God consciousness, you get to a state of an undifferentiated, the fabric of radiant light. But even then, you are not liberated, although you are in a state of Nirbeeja Samadhi (that is, seedless desireless state of ineffable consciousness).

That is the sweet nurse of nature who you know as Mulaprakriti. This is the final veil of delusion where the Yogi feels the "I-am-ness of the universe." Then he realizes through awakening that the feeling of I am all universe is a Veil of Maya. Then She Maya moves. That is the Divine Universal Mother, and unless she moves out of your way, you cannot see Him, about whom we know nothing. I don't call Him "God" or this or that because I don't know. The Universal Mother showers the blessing when she moves her curtain of the Ultimate Maya leading to the Ultimate Realization, so high is this state of Prati-prasav. the state of withdrawal zeroing in through the great star, like an infinite lotus. You have to pass through the matrix. You have to pass through the Divine Womb – the word matrix is taken from the Sanskrit word "matrica". So the correct pronunciation of matrix is matric. Matri. Padma Matrika – she is called Divine Lotus Mother.

So, you have to pass through the womb of the lotus mother to her Divine Awareness. When she moves, then you go into the non-being essentiality. The successful master and the successful disciple have already passed onto the state of the rings past not. Those who know it tell it not and those who tell it know it not. The master has died unto his disciple. And so many times have they died together that they have become deathless and immortal. This is the paradox of death. That when you die once, you die. When you die many times, you become deathless, and another name for deathlessness is immortality. And so in immortality is the successful story of the SatGuru and the true disciple. Where he makes the disciple realize immortality is Servant to Divinity.

I've taken you along the inner journey of the master-disciple relationship. He takes you from the atomic to the sub-atomic, from the sub-atomic, he gets rid of your protons and electrons and gets you to the electronic state, and then gets you to the state of light. Transcending light, you are taken to Divine Consciousness. This is the journey, the inner most inward journey of the Master's disciple. I know that you have never heard of the story before, and you won't hear again. This is inspired from within, and I don't think there is anything else worth saying after this. The Master takes you to the state of non-being essentiality – the state of aloneness called Kaivalya. You go to the state where your centre is everywhere, and your circumference nowhere.

Moses' Second Commandment As Understood By Gurunath - What is meant by idol worship as a Sin?

What Did Moses Mean, "Thou shalt not worship idols"? He meant don't idolize your perishable physical body which leads to ego worship. Rather worship the Godessence within you. I felt it absolutely necessary to clarify this commandment. Initially devotees must concentrate their minds on the idol/an object and then go on to the advanced Samadhi of Godessence Absorption within.

Moses said it long time back. The first direct glaring example is taken directly from the mouth of Moses who said God's words. "Thou shalt have no other god before me; thou shalt not worship idols. The true meaning of this is, do not focus your identity on your physical body. Shift your identity, and think that you are consciousness rather than this house of flesh and bone which sleeps, decays, and dies.

This is what he could have meant by do not worship idols, but much more esoteric. It means you should not identify with your physical body or with any statues of Gods and Goddesses but you should identify with your consciousness. With all due respects to one of the greatest Avatars, Moses, who I associate very closely with Sri Yukteswar, he should have explained this more clearly. He said thou should not worship idols, but it is not possible for anyone to not worship idols at the initial stages. You have to have an idol, otherwise how will you bind your mind to the object of your love? Once your mind is bound to your MahaGuru, it penetrates the atoms and then you merge and feel you are a part and parcel of Shiva. You become associated and integrated with Shiva. If you keep meditating, you go into the subatomic sphere, in a different dimension, you penetrate the atoms of being Shiva and go into the subatomic particles of Shiva. If you keep looking at it then, the form – the idol – of Shiva will disappear.

So, the idol worship will disappear automatically and then there will be what worship? Attribute worship. Then there will be no form – there will be just a bliss. He will be you and you'll be him. You'll become one with him. Samyam. And when you become one with him there'll be no idol worship. There'll be no form and then you will feel that you are floating in an ocean of bliss. Then you will be worshipping not Shiva, but the attribute of Shiva called Satchidanand. And then when you go still deeper, the attribute will disappear, and you will just be observing and being the whole of the mind and matter of the universe. So first, you'll be an integral part of the deity you worship, the idol you worship, then you'll be its attributes, then you'll be beyond attributes and become pure consciousness. You are immortal consciousness.

You are telling us not to do idol worship, but to do what? I am here telling you, first begin with the idol worship and train your mind to focus on the figure of your beloved. Once your mind is focused, go deeper, and the form disappears. Many of you when i give Shivapat, the form disappears. Have you seen that? The idol disappears. So that's what he means when he says do not idol worship. But that is an advanced stage. You cannot get to the stage of no idol worship before first worshipping the idols. Don't tell me the whole of Islam and the whole of Christianity can go straight into the state of Samadhi – the no mind state of Cosmic Awareness – can they? So I think he jumped ahead and you hadn't given to kindergarten the things of kindergarten first."

You have to idol worship to get to a state of non-idol worship. To get to a state of non-doing, you have to do something. This is the psychology of the human mind – that it has to be bound to a particular person, place or thing. It has to be concentrated, and then your concentration reaches what is called the vanishing point. You concentrate on a point and when your concentration reaches the vanishing point, the idol before you disappear. Thou shalt not idol worship. Oh Lord, I have fulfilled your desire and your commandment by intensely focusing on the idol, so that I made it disappear. I have entered into a subtler strata. From the atomic strata, I have entered the subatomic strata, where, oh Lord, now I am not worshipping idols – neither yours nor anyone's. I am worshipping attributes of the truth that you are and, as I go into the attributes, I still have the eye in me. I still have the proton. At this stage, floating in a sea of bliss, I loose myself, I lose my ego, and I am everywhere. I lose my ego at the subatomic state when i enter the electron. So I have got rid of the desires which is a neutron. I've gotten rid of the activity of mind which is the ego, the proton, and now I can take the final leap of divine consciousness and I rid myself of the ultimate building block of creation, which is called the electron. Once I split the electron, I go into he about whom naught may be said, which people variously call Samadhi or the Nirvikalpa Samadhi. But then too, I am pulled back again and again by past desires which bubble up from the surface of my mind's lake and pull the flying swan down into the weeds of desire, delusion and error. The non-idol worship of God as Pure Consciousness is the highest form of God worship.

How the True Kriya Master Overcomes Ego

When the Masters take this on (garland of flowers), they are not affected by the ego. They want to take this off and run away in the silence, but the disciple says put it on and you cannot hurt anybody's feelings, so he puts it on. It is an ego thing of honour.

In India, we when we are alone and we are in the Himalayas, then where is the ego? When the tiger confronts you on a lonely path, then where is the ego? And everything else dissolves with the ego. The fight - flight adrenaline kicks in and the ego is transformed to the adrenaline.

Ours is a small spiritual group and we are trying to protect the world from destruction. We are giving a technique of Kriya Yoga. If the ego affects you, then it kills the spirituality within you. You have to be very careful not to let anything affect you. Masters are such that if you put a diamond crown on them, they will not care, but if you put it on a person who's not developed, he'll think he's the king!! That's the difference between a Master and the disciples. They are on the path, and they must guard against this. Sometimes, even great people, celebrities and dignitaries, who aren't advanced on the spiritual path get an ego. Of course, there's nobody to check them and there's no immediate advantage or destruction, but it just increases the coating of the "I" – "I am somebody special, sitting on this old, special chair and I am the only one with the power." So, if you give it to somebody who's immature, then it's a dangerous thing. That's why we don't do this to people who are not that level get power drunk. I was objecting to this, washing the Guru's feet at the Guru Poornima Puja. but then the disciples, who have a deep culture and are wanting to express their heart's desire and to teach this culture which has come down for thousands of years, insisted. I don't think in my twenty years of teaching that I have ever got my feet washed. I would rather get my head washed and shampooed since all the best salons are here. The true Master avoids all ego inflating activities.

So this is the training to give them humility and love and honour. All of you are not just souls who have met me for three months or one month or six months – it's not like that. You have met me from past lives. We all have deep connection from past lives. That's why I never worry about people who come and go. We should not be too worried. We have done our bit. People have made their choice. Anyone is at liberty to go anywhere they want. Those who are connected to the Master from a past life face tests, and when they have to confront the test, then that is to show how deep they are connected to the Master. So it is a past life connection. Sometimes the Master gives something to open the blindfold. He behaves in a very weird way. He hits you with a stick on the head. Those who are deep will say "I know this is a test." So they carry on. Flaky and flighty ones will fly away. Doesn't make a difference to the Master. At all. This is how they deal with the disciples' ego.

Don't Be a Spoiled Brat: Spiritual Laws of Patience and Stress Relief

People always think that we are subject to the students. We are not. Someone said, "they're ready – your disciples are ready," and I said, "we'll let them wait." I mean, we have to wait for twelve years standing on one leg for the Master, "come Master, come." If he doesn't come, we keep waiting. That is the Guru-disciple texture. He doesn't run around for the disciple. This is what we must teach you, that you have to wait with patience. Although the Guru is your birth right, although you have to get the divine, you must learn the lesson of patience. You have none – you want it immediately. "I want it now, Now!" Instant gratification is now enough, that's how impatient the spoiled brats are. They must mature their minds by Satat Abhyas". They need to learn the lesson to be steadfast in their Yoga practice. And if they can't do it, they throw tantrums and they go away. Well, you are the loser, then, go! And these deadlines have been the cause of the destruction of the human mind and led them to tension and death. Deadline, deadline, deadline, die. Deadline, deadline, deadline, die. You see it in all these fellows, the workaholic CEOs who overwork themselves. The greed for money saps them dry. When they have the money, they find it's worthless. It cannot give the inner joy; they're missing the true life. They're missing the true life, because the stress generated by earning the money gives the heart a jolt and those earning are spent for the hospital bill.

I am the infinite Divinity, this body is but a speck.
Behind this body speck of ours, the infinite river of Divinity flow.

The Eternal Guru Principle Revealed

As you advance in meditation, the atomic structure of the form of the Christ or Krishna, disappears. Then you perceive the attributes and then the truth. So the form of God changes, but the consciousness remains.

Similarly with the Guru: If you depend upon the outer form, you will depend as long as you need to grow out of that form, and then that form will disappear. His attributes will become apparent – of love, of teaching you, of disciplining you. And even that will disappear in your higher states. The essence of the Guru will remain as pure consciousness.

Now if you depend upon these, the Guru and God, God is the eternal everlasting essence, and the Guru teaches the eternal everlasting essence and has also experienced it. He is the Satguru. So, both of them are worth it because they don't let you down, they take you from here to Eternity to realize the Final Reality.

In a material thing, say a Ferrari or some money or something, that thing is ignorant of God. So when you get a physical attachment, and say the Ferrari gets into a accident, your hopes are dashed and you get disappointed. They don't have the eternal principle. They're not trained nor evolved, whether animate or inanimate objects. Do you understand? So if you depend on any person, place or thing for your happiness - all things are subject to change.

And therefore, anything that is subject to change - when it changes, and you cling onto the past of what you like, and this disintegrates before your eyes, your liking disintegrates. Then you will be disappointed, you will be sorry, and you will be crying for that which is not yours.

So it does not apply to the Satguru, but it applies to material things: That everything is subject to change, disease, decay and death. And therefore, invest and love only that which is everlasting, whether it be in form, or whether it be formless.

In the Guru, the Satguru as a personality, being in the relative

world, aren't there always flaws in the personality on that level? Wouldn't there be certain aspects of the Satguru's personality that one cannot rely on?

The Satguru is not a personality. The Satguru is an individuality. He cannot be divided: He is complete, whole and akhanda. The personality you see is that you have misunderstood the Satguru.

And the Satguru is bound to mislead you in personality and train you and whip you and train you and mislead you and weaken you and lead you astray, and give you false notions about yourself and about himself and create a great ruckus and havoc. To make the boat that you are, ready to sail the high seas, if he doesn't prevent every leakage in your boat, you'll drown in the Pacific Ocean. So he has to make you well and hammers you hard, from without and give support from within.

So it is not the personality of the Guru that you look at because the personality itself means flaw. If we didn't have a flaw, we would not have a nose and eyes and look different. We'd all be a round ball, identical to one another. That's perfection. Right? But because this is a world of relativity, this is a world of personality, we interact with one another; we interact with our strengths and weaknesses, and we learn from one another. This is to work out our Karma. If you have understood the Satguru as a personality, then you have misunderstood him. That's your biggest mistake. So you have to understand him as an individuality, not as a personality; because personality is exactly what the Satguru is not. The "persona" is a Greek word meaning mask, facade, falsehood. The persona is not true. The SatGuru is Divine Consciousness you feel in your deepest meditations.

Masquerade – personality is exactly what Maya is. The definition of personality is: "That which appears to be, but is not."

When I connect my heart to your heart, what is your heart? Is it not your personality's heart?

You don't connect to my heart. You don't connect to my soul. You connect to the Spirit of my soul; and then you will not falter nor go wrong. In the Shivapat when I make you experience my thought free state of Awareness, I am introducing my Thought Free State of

Awareness. I am introducing my True Self to you! That's my Divine Heart.

Specifically, about the rainbow bridge that connects the disciple's heart to the Master's heart . . .

The rainbow and Heart are physical locations to help you concentrate on the physical heart and then yet to my consciousness with that heart!

The rainbow bridge is a steppingstone. These are steppingstones or meditation techniques. They are good. I give you those main steppingstones because everybody doesn't go directly go to the source. So steppingstones are good, but don't get hung up on them. These are just techniques. Techniques are crutches. When you get wings then you drop your crutches. The flower falls when the fruit appears.

So after heart to heart, then connect Soul to Soul, and then connect Spirit with Spirit. That is in Samadhi At-one-ment. This is important. So, our physical hearts are the outer form of the inner Hearts of Consciousness our True Spirit.

Does the Guru use his personality to manipulate the disciple to do things?

Well, he can "hit" you a certain way to release your blindfold. You know when the Master hits the disciple, or he behaves in a certain way, it is to remove the ignorance of the hands which cover the eyes of the soul. So when you put the hands of your mind upon the eyes of the soul and cry that you cannot see, then Guru applies various devices and techniques to remove the hands of your mind from the eyes of your soul so that you can behold the Eternal Spirit that resides within the essence of your soul.

It would be nice if you just told me that: "Don't pay attention to my personality - My Pure Being is Pure Consciousness."

When the right times comes, the Master tells the disciple, and the right time was today, at this moment, so I have told you.

And I have told all of you that I am not the personality; I am the consciousness. So what you must do is exchange your personalities and take instead your own individualities. So the Guru takes away from you your personalities – your mask, your falsehood – which is very painful, and gives you in its stead self-realization, which is your personal individuality. Which is:

> You're not this house of flesh and bone
> Which sleeps decays and dies
> You are immortal consciousness
> Lord of the earth and skies

So, you are Alakh Niranjan. And don't you say every day: I tell you, "Alakh Niranjan" and you say "Adesh, so be it Guru." And every day you're being told that you are not, we are not the personality. We are the individuality.

And the personality of the Guru will definitely play Ducks and Drakes with you. He has to be in the personality, nor will their karma be worked out! For him to do this in Relative life, he adorns a relative personality.

The Satguru Helps You Get to Supreme Reality

The Guru does not encourage any attachment or any love of money. The Guru encourages your consciousness to leave that money and that attachment, and he will help you to seek God and God alone. But if your money comes in the way of God then he will catch it and throw it out. Anything which comes in your way to God, the Guru will remove that obstacle. So the highest purpose, the highest relationship between the Satguru and the disciple is he sees that the disciples journey to God is smooth and unhindered.

SatGuru will not help you to get a Ferrari, but if each time you sit in the Ferrari and you go into samadhi, he will help you to get a Ferrari. Anything which helps you to get to God. Suppose every time you put on a gold chain you get into samadhi, the Guru will help get you a gold chain. But if you want the gold chain to sell it and make money he will throw away your gold chain. So anything which helps you to get to God, the Guru is with you on the journey.

You have asked me so many questions, but I have always kept to the same focus. What is the focus? What is the concentration? I am concentrating on one thing only. What am I concentrating on?

The Supreme Reality!.

Kriya Yoga Requires Flexible Discipline

When we sit for the breathing of Kriya yoga, the practice, sometimes we have a distracted mind. Sometimes we have a concentrated mind and we practice the Kriya breath. The Shiva-Shakti Anusandhan, Shiva Breath, or Pran-Apan Yagna – all of this goes by the name of Kriya Yoga. When we have a concentrated practice, we say it went well, and when we have a distracted meditation while we are practising our breath, we say that the meditation was not good.

Over and above, whether you have a good or bad meditation, the encouraging thing I want to tell you is that, if you just breathe regularly for one hour a day, even if it's half an hour in the morning and half an hour in the evening, whether your meditation goes well or not well doesn't matter. If you breathe regularly for one hour a day with awareness, even if it be a distracted mind awareness or a concentrated mind awareness, it doesn't matter, one thing sure happens. The ceaseless influence of the abrasion of the breath on the mind, refines the mind to crystal clarity. Even if you breathe in a distracted mind, it transforms it to a crystal clarity. The breathing itself refines the mind. And when the mind is refined., That means your thinking mind is transformed into the intuitive mind. That means Manas is transformed into Buddhi. Just by breathing regularly, all things set apart, day in and day out with awareness, your mind is transformed into an effulgent radiance. This is the beauty: the Genius Babaji said, "Let's breathe with awareness up and down the spine."

Every second is a waste of time when we don't think of the Divine. Why does He make us like this, flimsy and sloppy that we can't think of Him? Knowing the importance, we can't think of Him. If you cannot train your thoughts, you are not an educated person. You are an educated person if your thoughts obey you. So there are very few educated people and they are known as SatGurus. I am taking literally the word 'educate' from 'educare' which means to 'bring in the light', and the Satguru has brought the light into his being. Therefore he is called enlightened, and therefore he is educated. Not only can he bring in the light into his life, but transform that light in your life. How far we have wandered from true education! I marvel at this whole human error. Life is a comedy of errors and we live it as we like it.

You've got to discipline yourself first. A banjo cannot play when every string on the banjo or the guitar says, "Yay! I am free. Let me go!" with one wire going this way, one wire say that. No! The guitar or banjo will not then perform the act for which it was made. It was made to play the tune, and if every string of the guitar is undisciplined, how will it achieve its purpose? You have to be disciplined, and those who are not disciplined will wither away and the life will be wasted. So that it's not wasted, I am putting my life on the line to see that you are a finely tuned flute – so that when the breath of God blows through you, you play the music of the spheres and charm God and compel him to hug you. The ego of the people make them say, "It's my body and I'll do with it what I like!

It's not your body! My dears, you are not your body. Can you stop your pulse? No! Can you stop the blinking of your eyes? No! Can you stop your heart beat? No! Then, my dear, how is it your body? Your ego is saying it is your body.

Only a Yogi can say that, 'this is my body.' Can you control your breath Gurunath? Yes Sir! Not only can I control my breath, but I can breathe through your breath as well. Not only is this my body, but your body is also my body. You cannot control your thoughts and mind, so how is it your mind? Gurunath, is it your mind? It is my mind and your mind is also my no mind. All of you have experienced that, right? So now we cannot refute these propositions which are put, because you have experienced my expanding your mind to Samadhi States. .

Your thought goes into a blank. As a matter of fact, effortlessly if I am sitting here, you are already calm. The moment you look at me you are gone. That is the disciplining of your ego. A certain amount of discipline is required, because Ravi Shankar plays the sitar, and the sitar plays heaven. It's dancing and the world is entranced. But if the sitar is like the human being, it must be fine-tuned to its work – not too tight and not too loose. If it's too tight the strings will break. If it's too loose it won't produce the music it is meant to produce.

Like Buddha said – take the middle path which is not too austere nor too slack. A flexible discipline is required in the practice of yoga. Remember this: a flexible discipline is required and therefore when you are fine-tuned to nature's flows, mind melts into the opal glows. That's what you want. That's a heavenly mind. You can't have a mind which you can't control. You got your degrees from outside, but you may miss the main purpose you know. You fill the knowledge, you got your degree, but you have a leaking vessel.

> As a leaking vessel, never can fill
> the waters of life so pure and still,
> so distracted mind fails to retain
> wisdom's nectar in its brain.

So what's the use of having a leaking mind when you have done your Ph.D.? It's no use. The very mind must be refined to perfection by meditation and made leakproof. . Not the system, but the minds of the people who runs the system must be changed. Then there can be a change. I am not influenced by anybody or anyone – .

What I am doing is the real education – educare – and the real work. Therefore, it's your bounding duty to convince them, that they are off the track of true education. Before you die, you have to be educated. Let's bring in the light and be ushered into light, not die sitting idle . You can change your karma. The most important thing you're doing in life is practicing Yoga to be self-realized.

Awakening from Mindfulness to Soulfulness to Consciousness

In mindfulness, you are focusing on the image, and when you are perfectly in mindfulness, then there's no distractions, but it's only regarding the picture of Gurunath – where does he come from; who is he; what did he say at the United Nations – with no other "hey, get my coffee", "hey, let's go to Trader Joe's and get some truffle ... what are the latest fads that you guys have? ... truffle almonds?" So you get the distraction of truffle almonds. When you don't get those distractions and you're totally with one flow of thought only regarding the Guru – that one flow of thought of who is he; where is he from; what does he teach – that is mindfulness. You're not distracted. That is mindfulness. A ceaseless flow of thought without outer distraction is mindfulness.

Soulfulness is when he looks so much at the photo of Gurunath that the subject and the object become one. There's no thought then. I am him. I am experiencing him. That is soulfulness. That's a very high state of composed mind. I'm actually speaking about the psychology of mystical awakening – the psychology of spiritual awakening. Then you get to a higher state of expansion which is known as consciousness. When the mind leaves, the object of Gurunath's photo and Gurunath becoming one, he leaves a relative object – he leaves relativity. He leaves duality and goes into the singularity, which is not focusing on the attributes or the physical body of the person, but just going into his awareness, his consciousness, and fusing at a higher level which is transcendence.

So mindfulness informs, soulfulness transforms you into one, and consciousness is – it is eminent and is transcendent. It is beyond the physical body, beyond duality, so when you go into consciousness there is no thought, but the souls of both the people meet. In soulfulness, the subtle body, the intuitional body, meets, but the spiritual soul becomes one in consciousness. So, mindfulness, soulfulness, and consciousness infinite.

Yogiraj Gurunath Siddhanath

Part III
Discipline and Humility

The more and more I disappear
The more the self as God appears.
(Dissolution of the Cosmic Ego - a feeling of I-am-ness)

The more the I doth disappear
The more my self as God appears.
(Dissolution of the Individual Ego - Self-Pride\Vanity)

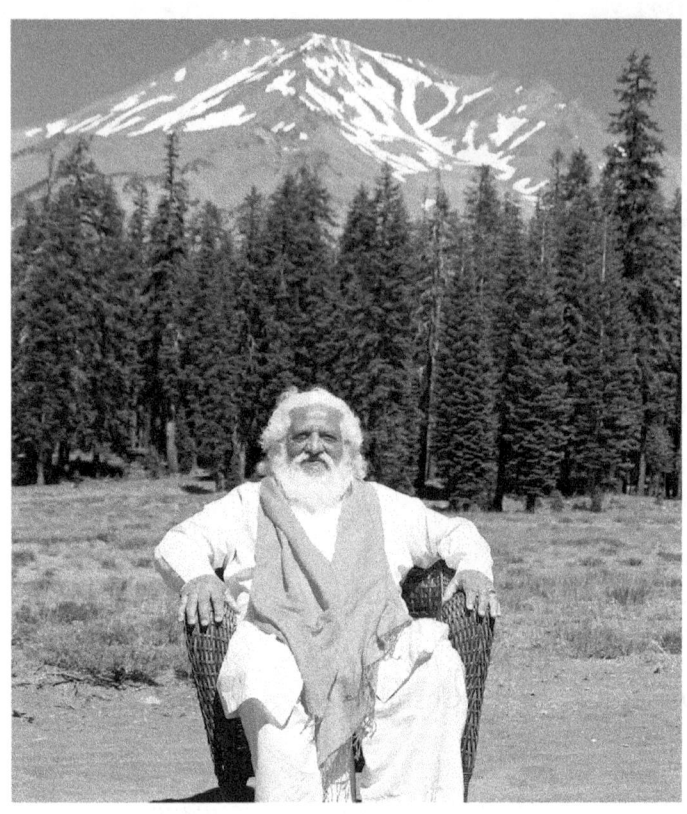

Yogiraj Gurunath Siddhanath

Service and Devotion – Shakti and Bhakti

Today, I am going to speak about two spiritual messages for disciples and what qualities they should strengthen in themselves. The first quality is the quality of service before self. Service before self and doing seva is very essential to dissolve the ego, because when you get involved in serving others, you forget yourself. And when you forget your 'I' yourself, you the ego deny. In serving others, you forget yourself and you diminish the ego. So it's a very wonderful way. That's why in all ashrams, in all temples, they do seva. Seva means selfless service – service before self. It reminds me of a very wonderful saying – a poem I learned. It is like a prayer. It says to the Master or to the Lord:

> "O Master, teach me to serve thee as thou deservest
> To give and not to count the cost
> To fight and not to heed the wound
> To toil and not to seek for rest
> Save that of knowing that I do thy I will"

So this gives the very selfless attitude to the person. By repeating this, you can cultivate the habit of service before self.

> O Master teach me to serve thee as thou deservest
> To give and not to count the cost
> To fight and not to heed the wound
> To toil and not to seek for rest
> To labour and not to ask for any reward
> Save that of knowing that I do thy I will

So in service before self, you surrender your will to your Lord, or your come into direct obedience to your Master or your Satguru.

The second message is about another quality to be developed by the disciple. The first quality is service before self. It is Shakti, and the dissolution of the ego by the Shakti. The second is the quality of Bhakti and Seva, the dissolution of the ego by Bhakti, by devotion. It's very beautiful, because when you surrender your all, it is called Ishwar Pranidhan – offering all you have to the Lord God whom you love, or to your Divine In-dweller, or the direct person who teaches you spiritual growth and evolution, who is your SatGuru, your Master. And you sing to your Master or the Divine:

> O Lord Let thy wish become my desire
> Let thy will become my deed
> Let thy word become my great beloved
> And my body thy flute of reed

It's a beautiful poem. It's not mine, although I compose poems. I don't know where I heard it, but I thought I should share it with you all. But it means that I am so in-tune with you, O Lord – let us say for example, O beloved Krishna – I am so in-tune with you that I am totally surrendered to you. When you blow your breeze through me, when you play your flute, let my spine become your flute and play the tune divine. Play your tune through me, O Lord, so that I may dance the dance divine and merge into thee sublime.

So these are the two messages – the qualities to be developed by the disciple: Shakti – service before self, and Bhakti – Ishwar Pranidhan, by devotion to the Lord, surrender your ego and negativity to the Supreme Master.

All my blessing to you! God Bless and God Speed!

Seva and Dissolving the Ego

So they asked him, "how did you get so much spiritual progress? I've got second, third kriya, you've not." He said, "I do one thing – Seva first, I lay the Guru's asana properly. That's all. And after that I do my first kriya." "Is that all you do?" He said, "Yes." Because laying of the Guru's asana is winning half the race.

You have to do the basics first – the Seva! We have not given importance to seva. Seva is a very important thing which the Siddhanath Yoga Tradition and the Hamsa Yoga Sangh has neglected for many years. Seva is a process where you do simple and menial jobs, like lifting the bench and bringing it here.

So what does seva do? Why are you doing the service to humanity? I gave the money to the Guru – I've paid my money. But this is not a business deal – it's a heart-to-heart. So, that is a very personal aspect which you should have with the Guru.

When you do Seva serve others, you forget yourself. The moment you forget yourself, you lose your ego. That's what the game is about. That's why I tell my disciples: you are coming to the benefactor's and you've paid the money and of course it's good – it's liquid Lakshmi and everybody likes the green dollar You must offer with gratitude and humility for your own welfare and your evolution.

If I ask you, how much Guru seva have you done? You have come to every benefactor's retreat, but how much Guru seva have you done? Today, did you help in the making of the Guru's asana? No! How much Guru seva have you done? Did you clean the leaves in front of the Guru's asana? When I ask you these questions, you will fall short on the devotional side. You are very disciplined on the Shakti side, but on Bhakti you are slack. You teach well but that doesn't dissolve your ego.

So, Bhakti should be more. Bhakti means devotion. In Shakti, you pay your fees, and you are disciplined. I like disciplined. I am more of a disciplined guy, and you get your blessing from the Guru. But on the devotional side, "Gurunath, I am doing my kriya. I am getting a good concentration. But somehow, I am not satisfied. I can't get rid of that little mouse which is running down."

> Hickory Dickory Dock
> The mouse ran up the clock
> The clock struck one
> The mouse ran down
> Hickory Dickory Dock

How many know this? It is a very, very philosophic poetry. I don't know whether the poet knew that when he composed it. It's the ego running up and down the breath, which is not letting you progress. You have to forget the ego. How can you forget the ego? When you are so busy nursing an ill person in the hospital or serving the feet of your Guru or doing work for your Guru, you forget yourself. That's the point – you lose the ego. That is the Master technique of losing the ego. When you lose the ego, you've won fifty percent of the race or more. I am concerned about your evolution – pick up the broom and sweep up the veranda. For others, it is demeaning, but from the Guru, it's not demeaning. Its illuminating for the disciple.

When Paramhansa Yogananda went into Nirvikalpa Samadhi, Sri

Yukteswar tapped him on the chest, and he went. He was glorious amongst the stars, and the whole universe, the sky, the birds, the trees, and the bees. All was him and he was them. And then he went in to 'The Beyond.' and he had extreme bliss. And naturally he felt that "my God! Master is giving me Nirvikalpa Samadhi – I've been promoted," which he was. Later, Sri Yukteswar was down there, saw Mukund walking around like a Lord. Then the Master's voice comes from inside – he says, "Mukund, sweep the balcony!" After Nirvikalpa Samadhi, sweep the balcony, wow! It's that sort of elasticity, that capacity, I have to have – to touch the feet of the Lord and yet be humble to serve, to sweep the dust of which my servants have tread on. So this is forgetting the ego – humility. That's why seva is important.

Whenever you get a chance, when I come to the ashram, many of you have seen the first seva mandal – pick up all the leaves in the ashram, all six acres. It sounds stupid. But in that picking up, people get so engrossed, like a child, that they pick up every leaf and they forget themselves. Every time you forget yourself, you lose your ego. You lose your ahamkara. Therefore, seva is very important and therefore this disciple who was doing the seva of Lahiri Mahasaya's asana used to be so engrossed in doing the asana. Of course, Lahiri baba didn't care for it, but now the times have changed. They didn't have to be taught, because it was in India, in the culture of India. Here we have people from all over the world and it's unfair if I don't teach them the protocol, and the devotion which you have to have. E.g. The most virtuous Guru Dakshina is offered at Guru Purnima.

Placing the Guru's asana, it should not be comfortable – it should not be too soft and cushy, but firm. It should always be firm, but not this way (sloping upwards). You are not giving the Guru abdominal exercises. My Hamsa Yoga Sangh, the Siddhanath Yoga Parampara, has the habit of giving me abdominal exercises, because many times not purposely, without knowing it, the asana is luxurious, but I am like this (sloping upwards). They are sloping down for the perfect posture. Even now you see this is sloping down and the Guru has to come to the front, so there is an abdominal exercise for the Master.

You've got to, in future, lose your ego by serving the Master. Lose your ego by serving little children. Lose your ego by serving the poor. This is the way of losing the ego and Bhakti is one of those ways. Guru seva is the highest thing you do.

If you go to India and you go to a place like Mathura, they serve you food, the seva, and in the service of that food, in the Hare Krishna thing also, they have carried it over and they lose themselves. In the North, if you go to the Gurudwaras in Anandpur Sahib and all, the people serve the langar, and the people who serve you the langar forget the ego. But the Gurudwara system is a better system since it's a double whammy – both get it. Have you been to Gurunath's ashram, where you serve the children? We serve the children. That's good. It makes you forget your ego. But we should do like they do in the Gurudwaras – they not only serve the people and the children, and those servers forget their ego, but in the end we who were served were made to wash our own dishes, so we forget our ego also. So this is a very, very good thing of Guru seva. Guru Bhakti.

Gurunath, there is also an incredible amount of joy that develops inside when we are doing seva.

Yes! But you see, Gurunath has spoiled his disciples by giving them an incredible amount of joy even when they do nothing. If I were a sevak, I would ask myself, why the hell should I do seva? What's this all about seva, when Gurunath is already giving me the joy? I am getting the great joy without doing seva. So why should I do seva? Why should I not sit in Gurunath's presence? It's not about the bliss – seva is not about the bliss. We all get the bliss, but you cannot dissolve your ego. The ego is dissolved by doing seva. That is the lynch-pin of the whole thing. So it's very important that you should be searching to serve your Master or to serve even other fellow disciples. You can serve fellow disciples. The secret of seva is the dissolution of the ego. There is no other way you can dissolve the ego better than by doing seva. Extreme form of seva is sacrifice.

I am curious to know about competition of seva, because one of the things I notice, not just in this ashram, but in many ashrams, is competition for the right to do the seva and this gets very tricky.

Now, that is a very good question. The competition of seva brings about a very thin, transparent film around the ego. Very thin – you cannot see it. Oh, he is doing that seva – I'll do more. He is giving tea to Guru at six in the morning, okay, I'll come at four. But that's troubling the Guru. What happens with seva when you compete is that 'I' means you look for brownie points. You look for credit and that 'I' looking for credit, that is the thing which destroys the seva. Instead of dissolving the ego in the waters of seva, that competition puts a water-proof film around the ego, so it doesn't dissolve in the waters of seva. So that little blob, it's like oil, it's still floating in the waters. So you have to guard against competing in seva. If somebody does seva before you, it's ok. Be natural. Competition in seva is a very dangerous thing, it can bring about a subtle ego, that who is more humble? Who has more seva? That itself brings about an ego and that competition must be avoided. Teachers have to protect against ego inflation much more than the sevaks. So, Hamsa Kriyacharyas be cautious, be alert! Kill the ego the moment it raises its head!

Last night, in my dream, I had a profound experience of gratitude and remembered why we have to come back to the Guru. Why am I here? It was amazing profound experience. Thank you! Thank you for giving that bliss!

Okay, so now I am going to ask you a question: why do you come to the Guru? Why do you come to the same Guru again and again to learn the same technique?

It pumps us up. It evolves us quicker with the same Master's vibration.

Okay, okay. That is a question of rejuven-detox technique. It rejuvenates you. It fills you up with the contentment, and simultaneously detox's your system.

It's never the same.

Right! Because our bond is with You. Your covenant must be with the same Master all along your Evolution. It's never the same! Every different cell in your body is treated differently, and unless there is the dawn of the spiritual sun in every cell of your body, you will not be enlightened. The Guru is dawning the spiritual sun in every cell of your body, and when you feel that every cell in your body is feeling like the rising sun of the new age – the New Nirvana Niranjan Moksha – then you are totally enlightened. It's very poetic. It's very nice. The dawn of the new age! The dawn in every cell of your body. A sunrise in every cell of your body – can you contain the bliss? You'll burst into trillions of sparks of light and merge into Babaji. You cannot contain yourself. If there is the dawn of a spiritual sunrise in every cell of your body, can you contain the ananda? Can you contain the joy? No! Then what will happen to you? There will be a supernova explosion of bliss. How do you like that? You cannot conceive that, right? And that supernova explosion of bliss will find you seated in the heart of Babaji. Of course, you will be just experiencing, but you won't know what is going on vis-a-vis your logical mind. You will know nothing. You are just there. This stage shall come to everyone. First things first!

But we can't start with a Ph.D. without the foundation. You can't start putting the flowers on the Guru's asana before you laid the platform. You don't put the flowers first. Doing Vishnu Granthi Bhedan is putting the flowers first, before making the asana of the Guru. There is a sequence. This is the sequence. Now I emphasize that for everything, there is a sequence. First, the foundation is made. You don't start building the roof of the house on the stilts, before making the plinth of the house. Right? The foundation must be strong. Therefore your seva must be strong. And, of course, some of us are not the seva type. I am not the seva type. I am the soldier type. I get on with the job and I get carried away with it, but I must remind myself that when there is seva to be done, I must do it, because seva, whether or not it's Gurunath's strong point, is very necessary for the flight of the Hamsa. Bhakti is seva and Shakti is kriya. So Bhakti and Shakti are the two wings of the Hamsa soul which takes you to the goal divine.

Then what shall I do, Gurunath? I am looking for seva and there is nothing to do. I say put your feet on your thigh and give yourself an acupressure. That is a type of seva. Do something which will take you away from self-centeredness. And it is very difficult when you say, "burning disease, decay, and death of mine. I am the lightning blue divine." So beautiful! It gives you a pure ego, but even that has to dissolve. So how many remember this technique? "Golden lotus am I, who divinity breathes". I've said that to dissolve your ego.

> Golden lotus am I, who divinity breathes.
> It inhales up with 'Sa' to open my petals,
> and exhales down with 'Ham' to close them.

Every one of you, when you are teaching the golden lotus, please use these words. You have to use them when you are teaching the golden lotus, because it says you are the golden lotus, but divinity breathes you. You cannot breathe a breath without his saying. This is one of the things which I told you dissolves the ego.

I said something the other day in one of the retreats. I said, "burning disease, decay and death of mine, I am the electric blue divine." You are using an egoistic phrase to destroy the ego itself. Even in this you are using the phrase – you are saying you are the electric blue who is burning disease decay and death. So you are using your ego to destroy your own ego. This is also destroying the ego, when you say I am the electric blue divine. 'I am' is ego. Maybe not an ordinary ego – it is the divine ego. But when you have burnt the disease, decay, and death of yours, then what remains? Just the electric blue. I am the electric blue divine. And if you keep saying I am the electric blue divine, the electric blue divine, what is the next thing the electric blue burns? 'I am'. Then you keep saying electric blue, electric blue or lightning blue, lightning blue. What's the next thing it burns? 'The blue'. Then you keep saying lightning, lightning, lightning, then the lightning stand still, it burns itself. It burns. When it transcends light, light disappears into consciousness. This is the way of, the wei wo wei , the skill in action. The action in no-action and no-action in action, where you burn the ego by the ego to get into enlightenment. First, you burn the ego by saying 'Golden Lotus am I'. That's the first way. But you are not involved. Second is using the very ego and you delineate light you become the lightless light. Where there is no light, there is no ego. There is no light or space-time continuum. There is no 'I'. So by the very ego, you dissolve your ego. This is a genius technique. "Burning disease, decay and death of mine, I am the lightning blue divine." And as you practice, sometime in the practice, I just go this way: "I am the lightning blue divine, I am the lightning blue divine, I am the lightning blue divine," no burning disease decay and death, because I don't see disease, decay, and death in me. So I go into next stage of Awareness and Splendour.

Yogiraj Gurunath Siddhanath

Individual Mind and Cosmic Consciousness

When I say 'Burning disease, decay and death of mine, I am the lightning blue divine,' there is another person who heard 'Burning disease, decay and death of mind, I am the lightning blue divine.' Both are correct, but 'Burning disease, decay and death of mind' has a huge cosmic implication. When you say 'Burning disease, decay and death of mine,' it means your immediate self, your personal ego, Your egotistic self. Okay? I have to make my own English words, because of lack of vocabulary to explain the thing. Egotistic means that you – body, mind and soul and personal present life – are concerned. Egoistic means the universal mind; the universal ego. Egotistic is tinctured with vanity. How many of you have heard of the tincture iodine? Have you heard of the medicine tincture iodine? It used to be given forty or fifty years back. When you put it on, it burns. It has a sting right? So the egotistic person has a sting. When he talks to you, he hurts your feelings. He is so full of vanity. And you see all of us all trying to struggle with the egoistic, but it's not tincture – it doesn't sting you.

When you say 'Burning disease, decay and death of the mine,' it means disease, decay and death of your physical body, your emotional body given to you in this life with your disease, your uneasiness, and your emotional suffering. Because you have to deal with it. You can't do the mind and your causal body disease before you do this. Now beyond your physical, emotional and mental bodies, which all have disease, decay, and death, and you can burn and prevent them from being diseased or decaying or dying in this personal life, when you say 'Burning disease, decay and death of mind,' the mind is a very, very tricky thing. It can expand from midpoint of your third eye to 13.7 billion light years across. That's the size of creation. So what is that mind? The mind is the universal mind field.

When you say dissolving disease, decay, and death of mind, what does it mean? Does it mean your individual minds? Or does it mean all the minds in the world? Because you have to finish karma with all the minds in the world. So that mind is the universal fabric of mind – the universal fabric of the mind field called Mahat.

After you finish dissolving the small mind of your ego, then you go to the community mind, the humanity mind, and the universal mind. When you dissolve the universal fabric of mind – that's going in to the Supreme, passing through cosmic star of Babaji. Going into the universal truth means penetrating and passing beyond the cosmic black hole, the cosmic Krishna Vivar. So that is the difference. This mind is dissolving the ego to get to self-realization, but the mind is dissolving the universal ego to get to God-realization.

The Prodigal Son Parable

Of course, Lahiri Mahasaya never told anyone "keep it up." Even if you did a thousand kriyas he would say, "keep carrying on, do it." And then some small girl would say, "I hurt my finger and I prayed to God and God came and now the pain in my finger is gone," and he would say "oh, that is a great thing. That's a great thing." So he is not letting the geniuses go forward and pushing the laggards up you see. This is just to give them encouragement. Because the guys who are advanced need no encouragement – the people who are advanced and sincere, they need the whip. The people who are lazy and prodigal, are useless country bumpkins, they need chocolates and sweets to encourage them along the path. Isn't it funny?

There was a father and the prodigal son had come back and the father had prepared a great meal and he rejoiced that this waste, this country bumpkin marijuana smoker, had come back. So the father prepared a great feast and the elder son went up to the father and he said, "Father, what are you doing? Here I am with you, an obedient child, listening to every percept. Every order you give, I obey. Everything you say, I do, and you don't make anything of that. Here this prodigal son, who is a thorough profligate, spending his time in drinking and smoking and womanising, he comes back, and you prepare this great feast for this prodigal son. So this was a very valid question which this advanced yogi had asked. This story is in the Bible. So the father, he replied, "my son, you are already perfect. You are on the path of meditation. But this profligate son, this prodigal son, a drinker, smoker, womaniser, wasting his life, has repented and come back again. So we are rejoicing and having a party. The son still couldn't get it.

The guy who is sincere says, "oh, I am doing a thousand kriyas." Okay, carry on. "Oh, I did one kriya today and I have left my marijuana." Oh wow, that is a great thing. The same Guru would say the prodigal son gets so much praise and the person who is already developed and advanced in Kriya gets no praise, because the policy is to give the advanced and the good person the whip, and give the prodigal son, the chocolates to come into the circle for the hamsanath mandala. To the fellow who is spiralling up to the peak, the Guru would say, "okay, come on, come on, you can do better. Go faster." It's like in running – you have a pacer in front of you because they are stronger. You have more capacity and in the end get the true wealth of Divine Realization.

How to love and heal others as your larger self

With relation to Kriya Yoga and Hamsa Yoga, how must we function and live amongst ourselves and in society? What should be the interaction? How should we be in harmony and how should we flow? My thought on this is that we are not obligated to humanity, neither is humanity obligated to us. It is an awareness moving down the river of time and we love humanity as our larger self and therefore from the fountainhead of our love, we serve humanity unconditionally. Not with any benchmarks, not with any timespan, not as a duty, not as an obligation, but we flow as the river of consciousness and in the flow of that love of the consciousness we serve humanity as our larger selves. Whether we serve ten people or ten thousand people is irrelevant. As Hamsacharyas, the spirit in which we do our work is important. Our individual present explains our individual past. We are spontaneously sitting here because we are meant to sit here because we love it. We did not come here as a duty – we came here because the good Lord has afforded us this genuine luxury of a spiritual gathering because he loves us. We love the Lord in every human soul and are therefore availing of this spiritual priceless time which we have been afforded in great joy. We come together as awareness in being.
The Siddhanath Yoga Parampara, the Sangh is an awareness in being flowing along the river of time, coalescing into a vaster and vaster consciousness. It is not straining oneself in the teaching, but teaching out of love to whoever would want it sincerely, knowing that the one we teach is a part of ourselves, knowing that we can breathe through his breathing and give our soul consciousness of a clear mind bliss to him. Like your Guru has given you, someday you will also give to another. Knowing that at the level of consciousness humanity is one, we serve humanity as our larger self. Out of no compulsion, out of no obligation, out of no duty, but out of love

Realising by our practice of Shiva-Shakti and Hamsa yoga that at the level of breathing and breath, humanity is tied by the self-same chord of breath – the chord of love – and so we flow on in our work.

But first let me caution you: we must make ourself strong. We must make our spiritual bank balance. We must be a spiritual billionaire before we donate a million we must be multi-millionaire before we donate a couple of thousands. So, we must make ourselves spiritually strong by constantly and ceaselessly loving ourselves. And how do we love ourselves? By doing the Shiva-Shakti Anusandhan. Selfing into the self by the effort of the self, we are strong after three to six months of sadhana. We continue to do that level of sadhana, that practice of spiritual growth, and simultaneously and gradually serve humanity as our larger selves.

Take little yoga classes, Hamsa Yoga and Kriya classes, satsangs and meditations, and that's how we work for the good of the humanity. Spread the work of God and Guru. Though your Guru or you may belong to a certain type or tradition, the teachings, let us remember, are humanity is one's only religion, breath one's only prayer, and consciousness one's only God. If this and this alone is realised to be the truth, then there shall be peace and love on Earth and goodwill to all human kind. The Hamsa Yoga Sangh is dedicated to the furthering of human awareness. It is dedicated to serve humanity as one's larger self and it is dedicated to making your life and those of others a celebration on this planet. The nitty-gritty of it and the details of it, you can work out as per your own spiritual inspiration.

Physics Nowhere Now
The So-Called Higgs Boson God Particle

When you come to the Satsang, or the gathering of a Master, you must adjust and fine tune yourself to be on the same wavelength of the Master and then and then alone you will know what he is saying by virtue of the experience you have, not by the words you listen to. Every word uttered is a transmission in a miniscule dosage, so that depends upon the individual receptivity. Behind the words is the living spirit of God. That is the spirit which has to be experienced. It cannot be bottled or subject to empirical tests sin the laboratory. It cannot be comprehended by the human mind or any mind because it is beyond mind.

Even God as Mind cannot comprehend God as Consciousness. When God comes down as Mind, He projects energy and the energy makes creation. From these particles of energy we think that we have found the God Particle. But this is the placebo effect. It's to give us an inspiration that if you can by the internal method of experience find God, why can you not find God in the material? But then everything on this world is God. Every atom in creation is God. There is nothing that is not God. So you don't have to have a special particle to prove that God was created from matter, because even if a particle is a God particle, it's still something – a particle has a form and a name. But God is not that. God is everywhere. God is nowhere. And God is now here.

Let us humble our intellect to vanishing point and get lost in His love. That's how you can find God. No matter how much you search for Him in the slush of mind and matter, you will not be able to find Him, because He is the very essence, so subtle and so beyond, that He has no particle, name, nor form. And yet he is the very source and substance of your existence.

God is not in relativity; he is beyond relativity and because of Him relativity exists. Because of Him creation exists. And creation is in God. God envelops creation. God is the source and substance of creation. But how much has creation realized God? That's what they're trying to prove. It is in relativity; relativity cannot reach the Supreme Reality, but the Reality can reach relativity. Therefore, God knows His creation, but creation does not know God through the intellect, because the intellect is matter at its subtlest. Creation can only know God by dissolving the intellect in all humility and merging into His Infinite Essence of We Know Not What.

We'll have to respect that. I appreciate the curiosity of the human mind, but I'm sorry, we'll have to appreciate that this Supreme Ineffable Isness of the Zero Not Zero is incomprehensible. But as energy, I'm prepared to call it the God Particle not in the supreme sense of God, but God in relativity, God the creator, Shakti. So the God Particle can be called the Goddess Particle, or the Shakti Particle, or the Goddessence Particle. But to call it the God Particle, which is beyond reality and creation - it cannot. You cannot comprehend, because God is beyond mind, and how can you with the mind comprehend the no-mind. The no-mind, the universal no-mind, universal cosmic no-mind, can only be comprehended by you going into the universal cosmic no-mind state. Experience, not with your mind.

You cannot fit God into the Higgs Boson God Particle, just as you cannot fit the ocean into the drop. The drop must die, temporarily, into the ocean. You are the drop. God is the infinite ocean. You cannot accommodate God in your finite mind, in your drop. You have to die unto the ocean and partake of the essence of the ocean, only as much as He wants you to partake.

So therefore anything which has a name and form, these are limited in relativity. So God in a relative sense you can say has been found – in the Shakti or feminine sense. Shiva cannot be touched. We just call him Shiva for name's sake; He has no name, He is beyond human comprehension. But you can say His energy, His dynamic aspect, the feminine energy, the kundalini energy, the Kundalini Particle, the Kundalini Bose Particle, the Goddessence Particle, or the Shakti Particle, and I agree with that, no problem. But to try to search for the Eternal Infinite and we lose ourselves. The ego is ever pushing on to think that it can bottle God in a dewdrop. You cannot do it. If He chooses to be there, then He can shine through.

And so you are suffering under the same delusion with the Higgs Boson Particle as a man who holds up a dewdrop with his finger and the whole sun is reflected in the dewdrop, so he says, "Ah, here is the God Particle!" It's not a lie, because the complete sun image is in the dewdrop, but is the actual sun in the dewdrop? No. So in the sense of your personal perception, yes the whole sun is in the dewdrop, but in the sense of Supreme Reality, the sun is where the sun is. This is the delusion of the Higgs Boson Particle, which they will realize in the future.

When God translates Himself – or works in close proximity to the universal energy – it is the Kundalini Goddess, the Mother of the Great Deep, coming into creation to wield and mould the stars and planets, and move Her energy of the Holy Spirit through every particle of creation. It is that energy which can create mass from zero mass. But the form is still there – the particle is still there. So it's absolutely not from the Nothing.

> This world our sages did perceive
> Is mind stuff materialized.

In relative sequence it is built
Deceiving mortal eyes.

So this is mind stuff materialized, which has been found.

All that is composed they knew
Must get decomposed
Where then does reality lie?
All matter being composed.

So also with the Higgs Boson Particle – it is composed of something, of form.

Closer to Reality is
That all pervading consciousness
of stillness through Eternity
Must of necessity proclaim Ultimate Reality!

Composed of nothing yet of which
all else is sure composed
It stands supreme beyond all dreams
eternally reposed.

And mind you, this word and poem which I say to you also is the shadow of the truth. It's just to satisfy your intellect. But that Supreme Reality can only be got not by the intellect nor if I talk about tons of books and information. It can only be experienced by the core of your innermost Nothingness, your innermost Beyond Description Truth.

Life is Nothing More Than This

People ask me, Gurunath, how do you develop your brains? So, I said, first, I have no brains, Secondly, I am only developing awareness. You see, there has to be some person who is called to total relaxation. Because the whole world, your collective mind, comes under the category of high tension. Orange level – you're not red level. But I am totally ice blue. Babaji plays with causation – space and time – like a child plays with soap bubbles. Life is not more serious than this. We've all been through the thick and thin of life. We've been through life situations where we've almost lost our lives, dangerous situations, but still, life is not more serious than blowing soap bubbles, in comparison to seeking God, your divine in-dweller. That's all life is, blowing soap bubbles. What you have to concentrate on is the Supreme Reality who goes by the name of God!

What is Your Source of Happiness?

The answer lies within, True Happiness has no Agenda. My personal source of happiness is the Divine In-dweller within me. People call it the God essence. And when the Divine In-dweller of a self-realized person, any self-realized person, transits to God Realization, then he finds the infinite abundance and he could want no more from this earth or from the seven heavens. The satisfaction and the illumination is complete. A contentless consciousness of total satisfaction is the source of all happiness.

Self-effort is the Key to Enlightenment

I do not believe and neither shall I allow you to believe this false placebo: that somebody out of the blue comes and he gives you a hug or puts his hand on your head and say, "okay, now you will be enlightened." Beware of such people, for this is a false placebo to deceive you and make a business out of God. So beware!. You shall be initiated into genuine techniques of Yoga when you come for the empowerment. I promise you; you shall be given the secrets of the Gods. You shall be given the closely guarded secrets of the Himalayas, but you should make your own effort and get your hard-won gold. You must have your own practice.

You train for the Olympics. It's not a comedy film, where you train for the Olympics and God runs the race for you. No. You have to run your own race and make your own effort. You will be given the technique. You'll be given the method but run you must.

Some people tell me, "but Gurunath, there was one yogi who touched me on the head and I felt very blissful." Then somebody says, "another person came and gave me a hug and I felt very blissful." And I asked them the question: Is that bliss everlasting? Is it lasting you constantly? No. But by practice of Kriya Yoga today, I am twenty-four hours in a state of bliss – twenty-four hours in a state of samadhi. Go for lasting bliss not knee jerk tricks which end in sorrow.

Of course, I do agree that my kind of practice requires more work. But what I am saying is, if you have the technique of bringing about your own happiness, why not be self-dependent? Do not depend on externals for your happiness, for the moment you depend on others – the hug of somebody else or the touch of somebody else, you'll become useless – a pulp. And when they don't give you that happiness, then you will be sad. Just like the usual stories – the boys become very dependent on a pretty girl or a date they like. When the girl jilts them, the boy goes into a depression because he had become a slave to that girl. He was depending on that girl to give him happiness through her smile, or through her hug or whatever. When she went away and couldn't do that, he knew that this is an insufficient thing. You get a deficiency. So I say in the practice of Yoga: practise your own technique, with your own guts. Create your own happiness by your own breath, which cannot deceive you till your dying day. Have a mature mind, don't fall for the immature demands of the ego.

This is all I have to say. That's why, although I'm a good Christian, I still do not agree to the philosophy that Adam and Eve were born on Earth and Adam related to Eve as a woman and they enjoyed a bliss, and he created the first stigma and sin with which all human beings are impressed, with which all human beings are burdened. Then came Jesus, thousands of years later, and he redeemed humanity from that sin. Now, in this basic philosophy – neither were you responsible for the first sin and neither were you responsible for the liberation of that sin. So who are you? A paper doll? A puppet? Do you not have your own self-esteem? Do you not have your own individuality like you create a sin have the will to dissolve it by meditation?

The original teachings of Jesus were that a man must live a simple life, not a hypocritical life, and by living it simply, by walking through thorns, by walking through good ground, by committing his own sins, by learning through his own vices, by creating his own virtues and learning through his own good deeds, he gradually evolves through his experiences and then comes face to face with his inner Christ, with the In-dwelling God. This is the practice of

Kriya Yoga. He did not take it the easy way. He suffered forty days and forty nights. He practiced tapa, yoga, and meditation to receive the incoming Christ. So also, you must practise Kriya Yoga to bring about the inner bliss within your own body. It's high time. Everyday you go to office, you come back from office, you're eating, drinking, going to the toilet, going to office, earning your money, coming back. Eat, drink, sleep, work, come back. Eat, drink, sleep, work, come back. So, this is a mechanical life. How about that part of your Jiva-Atma, your Soul? Aren't you going to do anything about it in this life? Aren't you going to use a tool, which you can use on your own, to bring about ease and order in your daily spiritual life?

It's not enough to say: "okay, I bless you, you will be enlightened in some point of life." Obviously, you're going to go, come to some person like me who's going to give you a tool to enlightenment. You'll use that process and you will get enlightened. But if you sit doing nothing, I don't think anything will happen. It's common sense. You have to make the effort. The alchemy of total transformation should be there. And this will not come by parroting a prayer in the church. This will not come by somebody laying on of hands, or by some reiki masters coming and putting their hands on your head and healing you. There is a temporary euphoria. There is a fleeting happiness, and that's fine, but what I'm saying is that you must make your own effort for eternal happiness.

If you take but one step to your Divine In-dweller, if you take but one step to God, He shall take ten steps towards you. And do not be discouraged if somebody tells you: "oh, the path of the yogis is very difficult; it's very dangerous. You cannot contact society. You cannot be with people." It's not true. It's easy. Anyone can do it and everybody can do it. And I encourage you to come and take the initiation of Kriya Yoga. It's not a religion. It's a way of life. It's about breathing. It's about you,. bringing peace and order in your daily life and realizing yourself in this life. This is very important. The sustained practice of Yoga meditation and the purification of the mind by detachment is the key to the evolution of Human Consciousness!

Yogiraj Gurunath Siddhanath

The Declaration Of Human Rights For Earth Peace

If earth Peace is to Herald the Dawn of the New Age, realize "The Soul Cry":

> **Humanity Our Uniting Religion**
> **Breath Our Uniting Prayer and**
> **Consciousness Our Uniting God**

To serve Humanity as your Larger Self by meditating on the Peace within and radiating the same to the World without.

Use the way of the Peaceful Breath which flows equally in all as a means for attaining World Peace. Thereby, diffusing Individual and International conflicts.

One's inalienable right lies in the furthering of the Evolution of Human Consciousness for World Peace, leading to the realization that your expanded Consciousness and Humanity's Consciousness is One!

By virtue of being a World Citizen, it is the inborn right of every Human Being to endeavor to attain the Consciousness of Natural Enlightenment for the Peace of all Humankind and exercise your Will-to-Good for making one another's lives on this planet a celebration.

As we evolve we live less and less in our bodies and more and more in our Consciousness. Hence, Fusion of your Positive Awareness with that of Nature's cultivates an improved and balanced Eco-System. **Help to evolve Nature with your Nature, because Nature is the Nature of Man!**

Allow yourself to heal and be healed of the negativity of your mind by letting go of the negative mind, which covers the Splendor of Your Soul.

Part IV
Kriya and Indian Philosophy

Concentration, Meditation, and the Power of Mind

When my mind is brought back again and again to the flame after being repeatedly distracted, the bringing of the mind again and again to the object of my focus is called concentration. Binding the mind substance on the single object and bringing it back again and again to that object is called concentration. When the mind stops wandering and is totally flowing into the flame with no bringing back, into the flame, then it is called meditation. And when the flame and the meditator are transcendent, there is no me left. I've become the flame. That is called samadhi. Concentration, meditation and Samadhi. Becoming the object in Yoga is called Samyam.

Some people try to advise me, to speak on Patanjali or the Sutras. This is the Patanjali of the Sutras. This is what Patanjali says. This is Raj Yoga. So when you become the object of your meditation, like in India there was a great lover called Ranjha, and he had a beloved called Heer. He knew no goddess but Heer, and she knew no god but him. So it was said that they had become so much of one another. They belonged to fighting clans – two clans that were enemies. But the girl and the boy loved one another, so they secretly met. Now remember, secret meeting is much sweeter than meeting openly, you know? Everybody knows that. When you have to take a risk, swim the river, or you have to do something for your beloved, then only is it worth it. If it's easy come easy go, there's no fun in that. So anyway, this fellow met her and he was caught by the king's men and was taken to prison and she was trying to say, "no, no, don't punish him. He won't come again, and I won't meet him again." But the king, the father of the girl, he is an unusually a cruel fellow. That's what history says all the time: the father of the pretty girl is always a cruel ogre. For the man who loves the girl, the father is the demon. So then the father said, "okay, come and give him five lashes." So Ranjha, who was big strong, was bound up and lashed five times. When he was lashed, Heer was connected to him, totally focused, and praying to God. And after he finished the lashes, they met sometime later. She took off her clothes and showed her back, and she had the five lashes on her back. This is the conscious ecstasy of yoga. She had become one with him, so she took his lashes. Neither did he get the pain, neither did she get the pain. It was taken by the Lord God but the lash marks on her back were proof of her at-onement with him.

This is the power of samadhi. This is the power of the Now, which is not a new word. This is ancient in India, as ancient as the hills. Called the Here Now Truth Alive. It's very ancient. We think it's a new thing, the power of Now. No, it's not a new thing. It is THE thing. Maybe it was his own realization, or maybe a rip off of the old text, I don't know. But this is samadhi – the Here Now Truth Alive.

> Experience of the Hamsa still,
> makes one know Divinity's Will
> in the Here Now Truth Alive.

The power of one's mind is enhanced by concentration. Now, I have given you an exposition of what is concentration, what is meditation and what is ecstasy. You are now in an advanced state of concentration. How do you think you get my no-mind? You are at that time in samadhi. You're so focused on me that when I stop my mind and become consciousness, you also become my consciousness. That is, you become the object of my consciousness. Do you want to skip my concentration and meditation and be like a post-PhD student? Be a master. Focus on the master and become a master yourself. Focus on me with open eyes and experience thought free consciousness an aspect of Shiva himself.

Three Great Philosophies of India

You shall be what you want to be, because this is a state of realization just below the Advaita philosophy. You're talking about a state of Advaita –Vishishtadvaita and Avaita Philosophies.

There are three states of philosophy:

Where you and God are different and you as a separate drop have not merged into the ocean. The drop is realizing the ocean and yet being immortal in its drop-hood as a droplet. This is called the Dvaita philosophy - duality. Then there's the Vishishtadvaita, where you will imagine yourself to be connected to God and yet be separate from God; your own identity will remain. And then there's the Advaita philosophy where the drop will totally merge into the ocean. Now let me tell you this: That a losing of the identity is a trick of the mind. The mind is the great deceiver. And it makes you say that when you lose your identity and your existence there is nothing to cling on to; there is nothing to identify. So it is an identity crisis we are talking about here. I want to clear this identity crisis from your minds, that when you lose the "I" – the identity – you do not die. When the drop merges in the ocean it does not disappear into the ocean, your limited Awareness of being is expanded to the Awareness of being the universe. You partake of the consciousness of the ocean when the drop merges in the ocean.

People feel it loses identity; this is a truth and a half-truth. The complete picture is this: that when you, the identity, the drop, merges into the ocean it does not die into the ocean to lose its identity but it expands to partake of a vaster consciousness without, with no ego, with no I-ness, with no individuality, but still the awareness of your being in the whole of creation.

This is the misnomer which I have cleared before and I'm doing now, that you do not lose your identity but partake of a vaster identity which you may variously call "God", "The Non-Being Essentiality", or "The Is-ness of the Zero Not-Zero." So this is the problem and this has been solved that you don't lose your identity; you partake of a vaster identity. When the drop merges in the ocean, it does not lose its identity – it loses its falsehood. It loses its materiality. It loses all that has limited it from being God.

But the awareness of its knowingness is still there in a more glorious and vaster truth. I'm in the birds and the bees and the stars and the trees. Yet I do not want to push others having it out. Anything that is selfish, anything that is decaying, anything that is segregating is destroyed. And everything is expanding, everything is oneness, truth, and knowingness. You'll have your centre everywhere and your circumference nowhere because you will merge into the knowingness of the boundless Being.

Look, nobody is forcing you to this evolutionary practice of Yoga. You can still be in a physical body, still enjoy your sex, and wine, and women, and laughter, and be yourself, die at the end of your age span, be born again and keep repeating the cycle of births and deaths. Nobody stops you. Go ahead. You're not born again and again with the same identity. But you're born, say, with a habit of drinking your wine every evening, and your habit for chewing gum every time you go to the movies. So those habits will remain with you and you'll come and – the collective habits – that is going to form your character. The sum total of your collective samskars, or your habits, are going to form your identity. Is that clear? And that's what you'll be born with again and again.

Your soul is in there, but it has the coating of your causal body, Karan sharir. Kya karan hai aap kai, punar janma ka? The coating of your unfulfilled desires – the causal desire. What is the cause of being reborn? That is the body, the causal desire of your body. Your soul body mixed with your passions and intellect form your identity. Your passions and you intellect colour the soul. The crystal soul is coloured. And therefore, this crystal soul keeps reincarnating. From the earth, the astral, the heavenly spheres; then heavenly, astral, earthly spheres; earth, astral, heavenly sphere; heaven, astral, earthly sphere. And so you will go round and round and round the mulberry bush of your karmic desires. So you can have that. Then a person wants to go higher. He wants to maintain samadhi and not to have these material desires. He has a higher desire: "Oh Lord, let me have the love quality; I don't want it to dissolve. Let me come again and again to worship you with love and devotion." So again you'll be born in the cycle of birth and death; you'll be come as a higher soul always singing God's praise, devoting yourself to God and this thing. And there's a third soul who will say, "I desire total immersion and none of this. I want to be totally one with you, Oh Lord. Then you and me and me and you..." Take out that book of Babaji; just read that poem: "Tied by the self-same cord, then me and you, there shall me none of me, Oh Babaji." So then, there is the desire of this type of person who wants God alone.

So these are the three philosophies, Three Great Mindsets: the drop is separate from the ocean; the drop becomes a sea and is connected to the ocean and yet maintains its sea-hood; and then, the drop merges into the ocean and becomes a part of the ocean. The first, the drop separate from the ocean is called the philosophy of Dvaita by Madhavacharya. The second philosophy, where the sea or the great lakes are connected with the ocean is called the philosophy of Vishishtadvaita, which was taught by Ramanujacharya. And the third philosophy, where the drop becomes the ocean and there's no difference between your is-ness and the essential is-ness of God is called the philosophy of Advaita taught by Adi Guru Shankaracharya.

People are born. They have a choice to follow any of the three pathways to Realization and freedom.

Yogiraj Gurunath Siddhanath

God is the Supreme Reality

You prescribe Kriya Yoga for a myriad of issues and problems in life. After Kriya, where does Ayurveda or Jyotish or Japa come in?

Because He is the Supreme Reality. He is the foundation and the Zenith of Creation and Beyond.

See, everything is necessary. I am not saying anything is useless – I am just saying, give to God the morning star. All other things are secondary details, that you can love them, you can enjoy them. There's Jyotish, there's astronomy, there's astrology, there's Ayurveda. Everything is nice, but you must put the divine essence of Reality within all these things. You must see through these things the essential unity of God in all the diversity of subjects and teachings and knowledge. You see what I'm trying to say?

Unite them with the thread of unity. Ayurveda is God. Everything is God. So without God's life, the whole universe lies dead. What are these scientists and all talking about, that you don't need God for existence? I think it's too audacious a remark to make. I mean, they're crossing the Rubicon here, going beyond their limits. You cannot challenge Divinity. You see, all these people, including everyone, for thousands of years, people have tried to prove God, and they have failed! For thousands of years, people have tried to disprove God, and they have also failed. Because God is not a subject of intellectual speculation. God is the fact of direct experience. He's the truth. And therefore, by the practice of Kriya Yoga, by chanting, we must experience Reality. We must feel its love and power.

Is Kriya Yoga More Advanced Than Vipasana Meditation?

Vipasana comes from India. It has been mispronounced – the original sanskrit for Vipasana is Vai-upasana. Vai means without, so it is without any spiritual practice (upassana). So it's mispronounced like Zen is a Japanese mispronunciation of the true Indian word dhyana. Dhyana went with Bodhidharma from South India to China and it was mispronounced as chán. It further went from China to Japan and it was mispronounced as zen.

The Reality of Kriya Yoga

India has tutored the whole world for more than two hundred centuries in yogic techniques and spiritual practices. So India is the source, and this is what is said by the great author Lin Yutang – a Chinese professor himself in The Wisdom of India. And it is also said by Will Durant – that India had tens of thousands of years before the rest of humanity practised the highest spiritual sciences and experienced the highest states of ecstasy and samadhi, which later trickled down and inundated the whole of Asia, and the whole world.

So, Kriya Yoga is definitely a more advanced practice than Vai-upasana, which people call Vipasana, which is the practice of anapanasati. It is again mispronounced: it is prana-apana – prana and apana – prana is the inhaled up-going breath that goes up from the base to the third eye and apana is the downward current that goes from the third eye to the base. So Vipasana is good – it's a technique from India we call the hamsa technique – observing the breath and just being. But now it's time to move on, so go for the more advanced technique of Kriya Yoga – the Shiva-Shakti kriya.

Is it more effective for evolution?

Yes, it is, in a sense, more effective because the combination of very unique evolutionary practices which evolve one into Raj Yoga Samadhi, if you ask me. But I would say that all of these techniques originated in the land of India. Not that India is special – the great ones just chose that country, that's all. It could have been Eskimo-land or Iceland or anywhere. Definitely the techniques don't contradict one-another. These techniques of Vai-upasana, Vipasana, and Kriya Yoga, they blend like the colours of the rainbow and they complement one-another. So we are not in conflict with any other techniques – we are in complement with all other techniques whether they be of Islam or Sufism or Buddhism. And you must realize Buddha was not a Buddhist, he was an Indian, and Christ was not a Christian, he was a Jew. So we have to get to the source – that Buddha actually practised the yogic techniques and not Vipasana. Buddha practised a technique like Kriya Yoga. Raj yoga and the techniques of Samadhi.

So yes, you can go ahead – there is no conflict. It is a smooth flow.

Origins of Tantra and Tantric Sex
According to the Nath Tradition

Speaking of the Nath tradition, is Dattatreya who wrote the Avadhuta Gita a part of that tradition?

Technically, no. The Dattatreya was a very high initiate of the tenth century. Some say he is an incarnation of Shiva, some say he is a manifestation of Krishna. He is an avatar and of a very, very high stature – totally liberated being. We have very scant historical reference of the Dattatreya, but he is very popular in the state where I come from, Maharashtra, so they have a lot of Datta tradition. They belong to the tradition of the lal pujari – the red padre – tradition and he is one of the highest buddhas, trying to liberate a group of people known as the Aghori yogis, who are indirectly connected with the Nath yogis, but are not in the tradition of the Nath yogis. They try to make him the guru of the Nath yogis, but this is misrepresenting the Nath tradition. There is no tradition of the Dattatreya – it is Lord Shiva as Adi Nath who is the supreme guru and his energy of shakti known as Parvati Nath – Udainath. Udainath then comes to Matsyendranath, Chowrangnath, Gorakshanath and the tradition of the great immortal beings, the great buddhas of compassion. The Dattatreya does seem to have been connected at some time or the other, but the true Nath yogis do not believe that he has any connection. Like the Kala Bhairava; Guru Data is the Gaur Bhairava.

I've always been under the impression that the path of tantra is also considered a path to enlightenment.

Yes, it is. The path of tantra is definitely a path to enlightenment. Tantra has its aspects: it has the right-hand path, the left-hand path, and the middle path. The white tantra, the black tantra, and the grey tantra. I do not know how they understand tantra in the western world here. Many books have been written about tantra, and many theoretical scholars, but I don't think they give the inner spirit. I mean, reading a tantra book from Abhinava Gupta can give you a totally different flavour rather than a translation from Georg Feuerstein. Feuerstein seems to be a person who's doing a good work, and giving you the outer shell – but that's all he can do, and he can't go deeper. For that you go to Abhinava Gupta or you go to the great Maha-Guru of Abhivana Gupta who started it. It was the Nath yogis who started it. It is Matsyendranath. Because before the great master, an incarnation of Vishnu, he says "I salute Matsyendranath my guru before I start this Kularnava Tantra" or whatever tantra Abhinava Gupta gives. I don't know if you've heard of Abhinava Gupta. If you haven't, then you better get to that book, because that's the source of all tantra.

You've heard of the Vijnana Bhairava tantra, where Shiva says to Parvati the Vijnana Bhairava? So these are two books you must have - Kularnava Tantra of Matsyendranath and the Vijnana Bhairava. Otherwise, your foundation is shaky. So please get to that and start studying that, because all these other tantras will come later, after the great Vijnana Bhairava which is the source from Shiva and Parvati. A lot of Buddhist tantras have been mixed into the tantras, but there is one problem with the Buddhist tantras – they cannot pronounce the Sanskrit words properly, so they cannot pronounce the mantra properly.

Tantra actually requires three things: a yantra, a mantra and a tantra. These three make up the process. So the yantra is your body, the mantra is the sound, and the tantra is the energy which connects the sound to your body. The mantric sound of the tongue connected to the yantric body form the tantra. So the mantra and yantra are necessary for the tantra. And there are tantras which can be done left path, right path, singularly, and with partners. And now there is in America started a new system, they call it the dyad system, but that I would dismiss it as humbug and bosh because America did not start any dyad system. The first dyad system was started by Shiva and Parvati themselves. Or Adam and Eve started it. Because the dyad system isn't a method started day before yesterday. It was started long back where two partners were used to evolve their spiritual selves.

What do you think of tantric sex?

I don't give it much importance. It's a way of life, so why make much ado about it? It's very normal; it's very natural. If two partners come together and they are agreed, why should we jump in the middle and say "hey, we are crusaders in the world and we are the only ones who wear white clothes and we have come to save you." No, it's not our business. It's a well-formulated science, and I think that the woman is a great power and an energy in the life of man. Just today in the television I saw that married men invariably live longer. They've taken statistics all over the world. Men with partners live longer than single men. That means they get the support of the energy of the shakti. The man supports her with his confidence, she supports with energy, and they live a more glorious and graceful life. It is more graceful to live as Shiva and Shakti rather than live as Shiva alone, or Shakti alone. It was not meant to be that way, I think they were born to fuse – he for God alone, and she for God in him. And a man reminds a woman where she should go, and takes her there. A woman reminds man where he came from, and a man reminds woman where they should go. So, he's born from her, and he leads her to God.

So, it's a cycle. So, he reminds her of the source as she reminds him of the source of his birth on earth. They're both right: the birth of consciousness and the birth of body. She represents the mayic aspect – the three-dimensional aspect of earth, mother, and circadian rhythms. He represents the Shiva and the consciousness aspects of the ultimate finality. She represents the phenomena of life, and he represents the noumena of spirit. And so the cycle goes on. Therefore, tantra is very good if done with the proper type of reverence for one another as God and Goddess, and proper guidance from a master.

Is tantric sex ever appropriate in the teacher-student relationship?

That depends upon the Teacher and the student. Why not? I mean, if tantric sex is necessary to have a spiritual child, one would have tantric sex with his wife who's the student. How's that? Is tantric sex appropriate? Tantra is a great science of great reverence and great depth. It doesn't even have anything to do with sex – sex is the least part of it. There's the dakshina tantra which is the right-hand path and the vama tantra which is the left-hand path. So in the right-hand path, they do not indulge in the process of tantric sex, which is the vama panth if the bondage is in witness of fire, like we have what is called a vivaha, atma vivaha – when you take seven steps around the fire and you take the seven oaths of marrying the soul with another soul. I don't think you have any such thing in America. You don't go seven times around the fire and take the seven oaths of binding the soul to the soul. That is known as the true marriage. So there are no true marriages in the in-depth sense of soul marriages – atma vivaha. They can, of course, in the right-hand path relate together in harmony and bliss, and produce a spiritual child.

The purpose of tantric sex, or any other sex if you do not want to waste your time, is to produce and have a spiritual child, which every mother would want. She doesn't want a hoodlum or a vagabond or a terrorist or, you know, just lying in the gutters smoking pot, you know. One lady came to me the other day and she asked, "I've left my first significant other, I'm looking for another significant other, and I want to have babies." I said, "wait, do you know how to have good children – children that will do you proud?" She immediately became serious. She said, "I never thought of that, but I'd love to have good children." You wouldn't want to have a demon, you wouldn't want to have a vagabond coming from your womb who would disgrace you and you would have to hide your face in shame every time, you know. There was the man who killed Abraham Lincoln, who would want to have a child like that?

So when we talk about tantric sex, be careful before you go into tantric sex. It's a deep commitment. It's not nonsense like it's been done in uninitiated circles. They don't know anything about tantric sex. Zero. You cannot do tantric sex unless your kundalini is awakened, unless the kechari is drinking the nectar from the head. You haven't even heard that these pre-requisites are required. And I'm not going to tell you in detail here because you're not prepared. You may overstress yourself or get crazy. So, the first thing is to produce spiritual children. The mother is so revered and so glorious that your head must bow before the word mother. She is the first guru who teaches us. All of us are here because of the one-word mother. America does need education, it does need tutoring to honour the feminine Shakti – to honour the mother. Then the second reason why tantric sex is done is to awaken the kundalini. Many a misconception has happened, many a wrong deed, many a deception. But it's human to err. So awakening of the kundalini and producing spiritual children are the two goals for tantric sex.

This reminds me of a saying which I like very much – a very natural saying. One student had tantric sex and he messed it up or something and he said, "it's human to err!" Then he added, "but it's so delightful!" So human beings are ever erring. And it's great because there's such a layer of hypocrisy in everything that is done. And everything about sex they say "shh" and everyone points a finger at the other person. But they do not know that three fingers are pointing towards them. So do not be a judge over others. Do not be a judge over others. Look at yourself, do not criticize others. We are all in the same boat. And if you criticize others and don't help them, your boat will get a new name – Titanic! We do not want a Titanic. Okay?

Could you expand a little more on how to have a spiritual child? Do you have to be enlightened to do that or can you just be on a spiritual journey?"

No, you don't have to be enlightened. That's what's being worked on and I intend to give that some time because I think that people needs this a lot. The society and the young girls and boys are totally going haywire with no guidance. Their parents are not able to guide them properly and hence this is very necessary, this guidance, to build up a solid society and give them a proper direction. And definitely great your strength if great your need. So long as the cry is ascending, so surely an answer shall come. For the spiritual child the Master Soul or liberated Atma will choose the parents who afford most facilities for the work of the Avatar.

Kundalini

Is sex bad for someone doing kundalini yoga?

When sexual energy is refined it becomes Kundalini energy. The mind exhausts you – it's unbelievable the trash the mind has and the way it comes out. It appears sometimes the mind is inexhaustible – it never gets exhausted, and the deepest vein is the lust for life and the desire for sex. That takes the longest time to exhaust since it is because of sex that we are here. We procreate and the animal drive is carried within our psyche for millions and millions of years, since the time we were amoebas to caterpillars to rodents to seals to whales to tigers to lions, we had this desire for sex. So that is the most natural desire which a human being has and he stills tries to repel it and think of it as a sin or something to be shunned. The hypocritical mind still tries to shun, and for this you must read Lahiri Mahasaya's book. Lahiri Mahasaya is an avatar. And he says, "sex came to me, I had sex, I felt good and I went into samadhi." Today sex came, I had sex, it was good. I am now in my samadhi. Finished.

It came; I did away with it. The householder yogi is beyond any of these things but some past lives' samskaras lingered and came up from the memory bank. It activated the hormones and the peptides in the human sexual system, so he said "okay, no big deal. It's come into my astral body from the causal, and now it has come into my sensual body. I will fulfil the desire, do away with it, and I will carry on with my meditation. So simple.

You don't feel guilty when you smile do you? Every time you smile and laugh do you feel you've committed a guilty act? Why should you feel that guilt when you commit a sexual act? Maybe because it is so thrilling. Every individual feels others shouldn't know about it. If you tell about it too much, you lose the fun – if you tell about your sexual activities, you lose the thrill of it, the sacredness of it and secretness of it

So therefore people don't tell anyone and yet, in the night, everybody is engaged in the same prayer that is the sacred of all the sacred prayers. One of the occult doctrines says that sex is the most natural and sacred prayer. But people ask, how could it be that sex is a sacred prayer when it stoops to such vulgarity and animal magnetism? The animal is natural and uninhibited in man in sex and it cures all the pent-up tension and psychosomatic ills

A man behaves like an animal and the more animal-like you behave, the more you enjoy sex, because so deeply rooted it is in your sum and substance. Yet we try to alienate our children – we teach them something different. We teach them that a stork came and dropped this thing the mother caught in her handbag or something and all the children say, "O we are handbag children – our mum just collected us. We dropped from the heavens, that's how we are born." Children must be educated when older with the right knowledge.

So Gurunath, how could we spiritually make use of sex? In the spiritual training for most spiritual benefit?

You cannot directly pull sex into spirituality because sex is sex and it's far remove from the high techniques you are doing. Just practice your Shiva Shakti and do your Maha Mudra regularly and it will pull the sexual energy and transform it into spiritual energy. During the process of yoga its natural for you to have sexual activity, after all Kriya Yoga was given for the householder Yogi.

Let your practice do it – don't mess with it with your mind. The sense of purity which you have during meditation is totally different from the carnal desire which you have. Always remember the saying, "the lily grows in a dung heap." By practice of Yoga the carnal desires are gradually sublimated in pure thoughts.

The most beautiful of spiritual people have been born through this sexual act, so please do not discard it or treat it as anything disgraceful. No doubt it retards you to the extent you want to enjoy the sex, but the problem is that it's so earthly satisfying that you cannot disengage yourself from it. You cannot disengage, because I remember one yogi told me he said, "Gurunath, I am a yogi, but please bear in mind, I am hormonal yogi." So, I said, "that's fair enough – you are a hormonal yogi." So, flow with the stream of natural life and transform. Ssublimate desires gradually.

I've heard it said about sex that if the chakras are opened up through Kriya, then the sexual energy isn't blocked and it can flow upward.

Purity of mind transforms the psychic energy of sex, not while having sex, but during your meditation and Kriya practice.

When you have sex, the energy flows downwards. But when sexual energy flows upwards, its becomes pranic kundalini energy.

I mean, that the sexual energy can be transmuted upwards.

It can be by Mahamudra and later Vajroli by your regular practices, together with purity in thought. Actually, there is no purity or impurity in thought – the thought they called "purity" for namesake doesn't mean the pot cannot call the kettle black. The pot is black the kettle is black both have to improve. So people try to degrade sex to lift up prayer and meditation, but it is at the cost of the Hail Mary or meditation. You cannot because it is from the desire or the passion of sex that the desire for God is created. If you don't have the fuel, which is the passion, how will you get the energy to think of God? If you haven't the energy to have the sex, how will you have the energy to think of God? It's the direction and sublimation of the energy that moves us to towards the Divine.

Just strip them of their colours – the emotion of sex and the emotion of any false notion – and use pure energy. That is called the alchemy of total transformation - to use the energy of sex bereft of its emotions, bereft of lust, and take the pure energy and use it for transformation. To use it for boosting your soul to consciousness. This is the alchemy which must be done and how we may strip this energy of the feeling of sex. Actually, in subtler planes, they both intermingle. The atoms, the photons, and the peptides are very amalgamated with the desire for procreation the desire for sex.

Behind the desire for sex or to enjoy the man or woman, the desire is to save your species – breeding children as much as possible, otherwise you disappear like lemmings.

Does an individual have responsibility to reproduce and preserve Humanity on earth?

This is a much vaster thought than you and I. It is a collective consciousness which has to look at the human race. And if the human race is dwindling and dying, we have to populate earth so that there is balance. This thing is just a natural thing like it would be for a lion or something to reproduce offspring. It is a very, very important bound and duty on humanity that it should keep itself alive. That it's a fun thing is a very minor portion of it. A sustainable society and a sustainable Humanity needs to populate the earth.

You can't say I don't want the fun thing and I still want to have sex, no one will have it.

What is the spiritual significance of marriage?

The spiritual significance of marriage is economical significance – that if you produce a child on this earth, you should take the responsibility to give it food, clothing, and a proper education so that he becomes a fine man in this world and makes the mother and father proud. Some offspring go on to evolve themselves and others by various means one of which is Yoga.

Like everybody would like to have a child like Vivekananda, like Ramakrishna, like Abraham Lincoln – even like President Kennedy. He did a great thing – he was the president and he made everybody proud, though he was the ultimate playboy. You don't want a vagabond or a terrorist to be born into your house, but it's not in your hands – you can only pray for the best and leave to God the rest. On the other hand, after marriage there are spiritual and yogic meditation and practices which can attract spiritual or great souls to the meditating families.

How is it decided, which Karma takes effect in a particular life?

Remember when I am talking about Karma, I am talking about the law. Of all laws, it is so deep and so vast, that even the Devas – the demigods and angels – go into a tizzy, trying to figure out: What is my Karma? Why does this happen to me?

It is the law of cause and effect. It is not just so simple, that every action has an equal and opposite reaction. No, it is not. It is something much more than that. It is something deeper than that.

Now the Karma which is already upon you is called your Prarabda Present Karma. The Karma, which has been stored in your collective unconscious is Sanchit Karma. Karma you make now is Vartaman Karma.

You have been born in the United States of America. You cannot change that birth. But an Indian like me, my Prarabda Karma has given me my face and form and circumstances for this life. I have to make it with what I have, live my life to the best. This very important to understand, that, when you make an effort to meditate by Kriya or get the guidance from your Guru, some guidance for the future, from your master, it is all to change and mould your Karma for the better in the future. This is to be remembered.

So destiny is not something which is very fixed, and which cannot be altered, as people wrongly misunderstand. Destiny is something mouldable. Destiny is something graspable. It is within your grasp and you can make your future, by improving your present.

You can prevent the effect of things from the past by practical application and precautionary measures in the present. And by meditation you can neutralize negative effects coming to you from the past.

So we all are here because of destiny, what would you say about that?

Because we created our present destiny by our past actions. Our present actions will create our future destiny.

We are here because of the cycle of birth and death, which was brought about by our unfulfilled desires. And these unfulfilled desires happen because of the type of Karma that we created, the type of action and reaction.

The cycle of birth and death is determined by Karma, our entry into this world of Samsara, our actions in this world of Samsara and how we go from this wheel of time, back to the subtle area. The soul travels from birth to death. It is propelled by unfulfilled desires of the past. Those unfulfilled desires present themselves when the opportune circumstances for their fulfilment happens not necessarily in the sequence the past karmas took place.

Hence, we are all the product of our Karma, unless some masters finished their Karma, choose to reincarnate again, pulling upon them the veil of Maya, the veil of desires, and deliberately being reborn for the mission of liberating of other souls. That is a different cause. That is a different case, but otherwise everybody is in the wheel of the Kala Chakra, in the wheel of time. And they take birth, are born, they avail of their Karma, they suffer or enjoy it, and then go back into the astral and causal soul consciousness. So, the soul keeps reincarnating, and your Karma, your destiny can be changed. The Karma and the Destiny can be changed by the practice of techniques like Kriya Yoga, Patanjali's Raja Yoga, meditation, and philanthropic works.

Doing your work, which you are meant to do, using your virtues to fullest extent and the best of your ability, the will to do good and be good, philanthropic works, and being good to your neighbours will all evolve you, and assist you in getting out of the circle of birth and death. Your present karma determines your future destiny just like your past karmas have made your present destiny.

In the Sanatana tradition of Hindu thought, we see that the cycle of birth and death is determined by Karma, and Yoga is the remedy to get you out of the cycle of birth and death. That is, the cycle of bondage. In spite of your not wanting a miserable life, in spite of your not wanting a certain vocation, you are forced to do it. This means the momentum of past actions has propelled you into the present reaction of doing of what you do not want to do. Getting a job which you do not like, having a life partner who you don't get on with, it is all governed by the karmic law, which is called the Triform Fate: the fate of past, present and future. You may partially change your past karma; you may not change your present karma and you can totally change your future karma under normal circumstances.

Now, being a philanthropist and being a direct practitioner of Yoga, both are evolutionary processes. Being good to your neighbour is also evolution. But in degree the rapidity of your evolution varies. Kriya Yoga is called the lightning path, because in Kriya Yoga the evolution is very, very fast. One half a minute cycle of Kriya Yoga gives you one year of natural spiritual unfoldment. This is the speed of Kriya Yoga.

Kriya Yoga is always practised with concentration and breath in the Sushumna Nadi, that is in the Sushumna channel of your spine. And this gives you the fastest evolution, the lightning path.

So Gurunath, if someone is currently practising Kriya Yoga and they go to a fortune teller, will the fortune take into consideration the fact that they're doing Kriya?

He will definitely take in the fact that you're doing Kriya. I have been to...I like to go to fortune tellers and you know, astrologers... and the Gyan avatar Sri Yukteswar himself who knew cosmic astrology and he said don't be totally a slave to it, don't depend on it totally, but use it as a guideline. So when I went the first time, they told me that I was practising Kriya Yoga, and they addressed me in a particular way. When I went to the fortune teller, the nadi jyotish, the next time, they told me I was practising more and addressed me in a more respectful way. Names change, titles change, so there's a constant updating, if you practice meditation and Yoga. There's a constant updating of your spiritual progress. There's a constant updating in the nadi reading of your circumstances.

And it is said, yes, like I've said in my poem, "Your individual present explains your individual past, to each one is allotted his exact and proper task, to the truth is truth begot, the liar gets his own, so do such deeds, do such actions, whose reactions you don't moan." So it's very, very important to thoughtfully practice with those activities, those thoughts which bring about good and joyous results. If you think of negative thoughts, if you think you're depressed, I'm a poor contrary creature and I'm suffering all the while and I'm all wretched and my back's paining, my neck's paining, my head's paining, if you go to all these things, then that collective thought, if you dwell on a thought of disease, disease shall be the outcome. If you dwell on the thought of light and love, light and love shall be the outcome. As yogavatar Lahiri Mahasaya and Guatama Buddha both said, "You are what you think." Which now the western world is taking up and they are making little notes and little booklets on things and thoughts which are true. But people are still demonstrating it in India.

What is Shaktipat?

It's an electromagnetic transmission of force which cleanses body-mind and assisting the evolution of consciousness. So, if your mind is perfected, you are able to release your prana and heal others. But you do not do any healing practices, I do not encourage it at all. I do not encourage millionaires to donate a million in healing. I tell them, unless you're a billionaire, don't donate a million. Otherwise, you'll be bankrupt. If you have twenty million and you donate one million, you can't break even in the cycle of spiritual progress. Only if you're a billionaire and you donate a million, then the cycle, the spiritual economic cycle can work unhindered. So, to do healing, you must be a billionaire to give a million, not a millionaire to give a million. You understand what I'm saying? So, six hours of meditation practice, half an hour of healing, fine. Three hours of meditation practice and one hour of healing, bad. I know I'm cutting it high and sharp because I want to discourage you from frittering away the energies of your mind. Do not fritter away the energies of your mind. Focus them and preserve them. And use the precious energies and vibrations of your mind to penetrate and pierce them through your lotus shrines to get to Satchitananda, the Divine Indweller. That's what it is meant to be applied to.

Yogiraj Gurunath Siddhanath

Train the Subconscious with Mantra

Focus the energies of your mind on God. You may ask me, "How can we do this, it's very difficult. Gurunath, we cannot do this, how can we for twenty-four hours think of God? We would love to, but we can't." Why? Because of the habit of past samskaras, the habit of your past. You cannot constantly think of God. But by repeated effort, repeated willpower, if you say "Ommmm, rhing rhang rhaksha rhaksha goraksha, om rhing rhang rhaksha rhaksha goraksha, om rhing rhang rhaksha rhaksha goraksha" day in and day out, then every morning when you get up, the mantra will automatically start in your subconscious mind in spite of you not wanting to do it. Now that is a true training of your subconscious mind – training it to do what you want it to do. Impressing the thought-form of the mantras on your mind stuff (Chitta).

So repetitive practice and perseverance in Yoga or mantras is the secret of success. The West never understood this, and they used to say, "We do not know…we went to India…," many people came to India, tourists and all from other countries, from western countries, and they said, "the Indian people do a strange thing. It's called muttering. They mutter. And what is this muttering all about? And they keep muttering for hours together." Then they found that muttering…now America is very educated and they call it the "mantra." And they say that "mantra" can reduce your karma. They have learned this and they themselves now have the malas, but while they were willing to learn, the time was not ripe. The time is now ripe, so people come and they learn their mantra and they mitigate their negative karma.

Because when you go to an astrologer or a nadi, the important thing that they tell you is, they say, "practice the mantra for the Moon, because the Moon is debilitated" or "practice the mantra for Jupiter or Mars" and then they give a mantra. Or the guru gives you the mantra, he is the one who has the authority. If he gives you the mantras of Mars or Mercury, and your Mercury or your Mars is in a malefic aspect to your activities, then that malefic aspect of your activities is mitigated by the practice of the mantra.

Now Kriya Yoga is such a beautiful process that when you breathe God through your spine, when you concentrate on God and breathe through your spine, that is the time the negative vibrations, the DNA in your spine is dissolved of its negative vibrations. So therefore, the practice of Kriya Yoga is most effective and it is called the lightning path. How do we determine and how do we know that we are practising Kriya Yoga correctly? One of the great hallmarks of the original Kriya Yoga is that it is practiced with concentration, breathing in your Sushumna spinal canal. So Sushumna breathing is Kriya Yoga. When you practice the concentrated breath called the practice of life-force energy in the central channel of the spine, you are practising Kriya Yoga.

Intuition, Psychicism, and Ego
The Limitations of Interpreting Astrology

There are a lot of people who go to astrologers. There is an Indian system of astrology called the Nadi Jyotish. Now, I want to make something clear from my side of it and let us start with the Nadi Jyotish reader first. I know those people – they come to my ashram. The Nadi Jyotish is said by very, very great Rishis and Masters and Sages of the fire mist, and they cannot be wrong, but people who read them are, more often than not, always wrong. The reason for this is they do not have the capacity to withhold the voltage and the message of the Sages of the fire mist. And therefore, I told the Nadi Jyotish people, I said "now look you're telling someone you're the son of Christ, you're the Gurus' father, you're the Guru's brother. You should hold your tongue. This is not your prerogative to say it." In Tamil, one sentence can be translated in three different ways. In the Tamil language, they will say, "Oh I'm your brother," but 'brother' could be of the same brotherhood. It could mean you're a Hamsa Kriya Yogi and not blood brother.

So, these mistakes are bound to occur and this I said to an immature crowd – a sincere and generous crowd, but spiritually immature. Nadi Jyotish is real in the highest sense – to contact the Nadi and to be in touch with sages like Vishwamitra and Agastya and Bhrigu and all these people. So, all people go to the Nadi Jyotish and they get their Nadis read. The readers of the Nadi Jyotish sometimes are normal fellows – they go out for a casual booze, get drunk and come back. They're simple Tamil boys. Some fellows do their puja – they're good people, but they do puja. I said, you cannot read the Nadi Jyotish with doing puja – you have to do Kriya Yoga and meditate. I said, "till you do that, your readings will be sixty percent right and forty percent wrong. If you want eighty percent right and twenty percent wrong, you must do Kriya Yoga. So a lot of misunderstanding has accrued from the reading of astrology, astronomy, and all these various things.

Even I have been to them, and they have also told me, but I never step out on it and never say I am this or that. Least of all, I never write it in my book. Maybe I was, but this would create a misunderstanding in the minds of the people. So, my message is don't go overboard. Because many ladies I've met they say, "I'm Durga. I was riding on a tiger, and I was flying in the air." Another one says, "I'm Cleopatra" and then, there were so many Cleopatras that I had a meeting of Cleopatras. I made them all meet. And mind you they were all beautiful – all Cleopatras, mind you.

I am speaking about this because it could be a very sensitive subject. When you look at a chart or you say something – whether it's astrology or whether it's Nadi – we must be very careful about connecting relationships. This could create a misunderstanding, or lead to disgrace of somebody. If it's put in a particular book, it could create a chain of misunderstandings. Therefore, the translator of the reading should be generic in his reading, and not particular. Saying that you were Jesus, or another was Judas, or you are so and so and you are connected to this chap's wife in a past life, this is nonsense. It cannot be read in a chart because that is due to psychicism which happens and psychicism is not always correct because it is grounded in relativity. This is another thing which we have to take up – that many people feel that they were El Cid or they were Davy Crockett or they were so and so. I will tell you what this is. Psychicism is a mixed feeling of intuition and desire, and your desires can warp your psychicism. Because everybody wants to be Christ; everybody wants to be Virgin Mary, don't you? And what's wrong in it? But the wrong thing in it is not your desire. The wrong thing in it is that you're feeling your ego to be what you are not. You're feeling your ego to be what you are not. And therefore as a Guru and a Sat Guru it's my duty to guide you onto the proper path. Psychicism is when you are in your emotional body, you have desires, and flashes of intuition come, but they get refracted in the waters of your emotion. This is what happens with psychicism – sometimes you hit the spot when you connect with the higher intuition, but if you mix it up with your emotions, more often than not psychicism leads to mal-information. The information appears to be what it is not. And therefore, you should be very careful of psychicism. There are many psychics – they read the crystal ball, they read this, that and the other, but you cannot in your readings pair somebody off as somebody's wife and somebody as someone's husband. There is a wrong reading and this. I must warn all the astrologers and nadi readers – do not to do this because, more often than not, you're wrong, and it leads to a lot of misunderstanding and disgrace. Maybe praise for one, but disgrace for another. And who are you to decide? Who are you to say, that you have such a power and authority?

So, this is creeping in to the system, where people have a grandiose feeling that they should be something. You are special. You are Kriya Yogis – you are special for what you are. But you have to see that one reading, even if it's one hundred percent confirmed, is holographic – it affects many different people in many different ways. And this trend has to be corrected. I am surprised why they don't come to me and check it up. None of my disciples have come and checked it up, because they were scared that Gurunath will burst their bubble.

So, psychicism is at the material level where your fluid emotions are mixed with flashes of intuition, and the emotions distort the message and the image as to who you are. Sometimes it can be correct; many times, it can be wrong. Now, clairvoyance is different to psychicism. When you are in clairvoyance, you are not in your emotions. You are already in a state of Savikalpa samadhi or composed Dhyan. This does not distort the image, so in clairvoyance, you can see things as they are. You can clearly see the image of a ghost, of a spirit, or the aura. So clairvoyance is developed by regular practice of Kriya Yoga, by regular pranayama, and by pure diet. Clairvoyance is distinct and specific, where astral vision is more dominant, in psychicism astral feeling is more predominant.

Then you have something which is called precognition or premonition. Precognition is when, by the virtue of clairvoyance, if you make clairvoyance dynamic, you can see an event before it happens. So that's precognition. For precognition, you have to be in a state of Samadhi, otherwise it doesn't happen, because precognition is raising your consciousness to the causal level. When you raise your consciousness from the physical to the causal level, you're seeing past, present, and future. You're seeing the Now. I'll give you a simple example: I am sitting on top of the coconut tree in Timbuktu and you're sitting far below, and you people are saying,

"Oh, when is our transport coming? When is my camel going to come? When is my bullock cart going to come?" I can see the bullock cart one mile away coming raising dust, but you're sitting on the floor, and you cannot see it – your vision is not there. I raise my consciousness to that height where I can see farther – I can see it further at the causal level. To raise yourself to the causal level is a steady state of Savikalpa samadhi. So, precognition is rare, but it is not an impossible thing. And in precognition, you can see spirits and ghosts. In psychicism, you feel you go to a spot and your hair stands on end, so you know it's haunted – it's got ghosts and ghouls and devils. It's very eerie, so that's a haunted place.

These things have to be understood and put in their proper place, so that we don't have a false notion of what we are doing and then fall in the ditch. Because many people say many things and there's not enough study behind it. People say "oh this person, oh he is a great soul and he's taken on the karma of many people – that's why he's suffering." Now, this has to be clarified. It's very educational. People need to know it's not bursting your bubble or making you anything lower or higher. What do you mean by taking karma? Do you know what you're talking about? That means you have completely finished your own karma and out of compassion have been sent by the higher forces, to go down in compassion and take the karma of other people. That means you're no less than an Avatar. And you're no less than in Nirvikalpa samadhi. So gentlemen, anybody taking karma for you all is out of the question. First deal with your own karma. I'm saying this very specifically, I don't see anybody who's taking anybody else's karma. And if I'm doing that I don't say it. I don't flout it; it's just there. It'll be made evident to you: Gurunath you came to me in my dream, you resolved it and you took away my karma, it actually goes away. But there's one Master. There cannot be two Masters at the same place – two Sat Gurus. It is the Master who is bearing the brunt and taking away the karma, so you have to be in Nirvikalpa samadhi to take somebody's karma. You have to be an Avatar. This is very, very important, otherwise the karma are not taken away. Sri Yukteswar took the karma of Paramhansa Yogananda and burnt in the severe fire of that karma. So are we all Yukteswar? No. So, we cannot take the karma of other people. This is an educational thing. I may burst your bubble temporarily, I may take out the rotten tooth now, but later you'll be happy that you were guided. It's good to eat the humble pie. Sit on the floor and be a normal human being. Practice Kriya Yoga hard, with simplicity, and Babaji will bless you. Babaji has the karma of the universe.

We're all humble people – we are not special. Even when astrologers have told me, I still don't put it in the book. It is for people to see and know and realize for themselves. This is very important.

Even Jesus could not take the karma of the whole world (note: this is the background karma of the world, not that of individuals) at that time. He took the karma of the selected few – all the people who had faith and followed him and followed the precepts. He did take a large amount of karma, but not of the whole world. It was a different story with Shakyamuni – the Buddha. Jesus was the bodhisattva; Gautam was the Buddha. Therefore, Gautam, the light of the world, did take on the karma of the whole world. It's time to teach truth, not religion. The Christ does take the karma of the whole world, Jesus does not. Lahiri Mahasaya does, Yukteswar does, and the Lord Christ, the eternal principal, is ever taking on the karma of the world. The future second advent, the Kalki Avatar, also does. But dear souls, you are not the Kalki Avatar. Neither are you the other horseman of the apocalypse. Leave it to them, rest in peace. It's not bad to be humble. It's not bad to be a human being. Don't feel bad – you don't have to be an Avatar. I always call myself a servant of humanity – a server of humanity.

It's very important to eat the humble pie. But you'll be shocked at yourself. When you're really at your peak – your peak of anger, your peak of jealousy – you tolerate nobody else before your sight. The ego can go to such extremes that it makes you ashamed of yourself later: "oh, how could I have done such a thing!? I didn't say that." But jealousy cuts sharper than the sharpest knife, and the transformation of jealousy and the thirst for name and fame should be reduced because it's the ego that comes in the way of your spiritual progress. So, beware.

How Can We Accomplish Anything While Wanting To Merge With Nothing?

Nobody at the present moment wants to merge with Nothing of Pure Awareness. If we had wanted to merge with Nothing, we would be Nothing, and have no desires and be total absolute lightless light and space-less space. So we are not at that stage as yet. We want desires and therefore, being in a world of relativity, we fulfil our desires.

As we fulfil our desires and practise Kriya Yoga simultaneously, our subsequent desires become subtler and subtler and subtler until we have no desires. Then we go to a state of Apara Vairagya after many lifetimes. And then we get to the state where we are poised to go into the great Truth, the Reality So it's a stage-by-stage progress to the Divine.

During our evolutionary journey, we definitely want to spread the message of Babaji. We want to serve humanity. We have compassion. Even the Avatars have pulled the veil of Maya and karma upon themselves and interacted with Humanity to push them along the evolutionary path. We want to save our brothers and sisters, and fathers and mothers from the quagmire of materialism. But when we get to the stage where we have nothing to do, we get to Vairagya, total non-attachment. It is a state of Nivritti – non-attachment to the objects of the senses. After which, we get to the absolute desire-less-ness, not even wanting God. Then God puts us to His heart and takes us close. That's how it goes, step-by-step to merge into the incomprehensible Reality!

What is true education?

Education comes from the word 'Educare' - to bring in the light. True education is knowing the essence of your true being. Academic education for worldly vocations and livelihood and the wisdom education for inner spiritual growth called Atmavidya. The education for spiritual evolution of Omniscience, Omnipresence and Omnipotence the Divine Virtues.

What is the process of death? What causes you to reincarnate and as what being?

The state of death is just casting your physical body away when it's worn out. Like changing a car when it's outlived its utility, then buying a new car. So, when the body garment gets worn out, the soul leaves it, drops it and enters into the transmigratory phase and is born into a new body through the process of reincarnation. The wheel of reincarnation is turned by unfulfilled desire. If the desire is unfulfilled that means there's attachment. If there's desire and you forget about it, you don't reincarnate. So the Kala Chakra, the wheel of time, is propelled by unfulfilled desires. Those unfulfilled desires which you have in this life and cannot be fulfilled are the seed which propel you to a birth in your next life which offer circumstances where those desires can be fulfilled. So it is unfulfilled desires which turns the karmic wheel. In Indian philosophy we have two main things: first is Karma, the law of cause and effect, also called the law of retribution. That every action has an equal opposite reaction. A person cannot be free from reincarnation unless all his Karmas are fulfilled. And the second principle is the law of reincarnation. As long as you have unfulfilled desires, you will keep reincarnating on Earth to fulfil your desires, and go to this particular plane to fulfil those desires in the emotional sphere, the mental sphere. And so this is the cycle of birth and death. And you incarnate in circumstances where, as a person, those desires will be fulfilled.

> Your individual present explains your individual past.
> To each one is allotted his exact and proper task.
> To the truth is truth begot, the liar gets his own.
> So do such actions whose reactions you don't moan.

You know because I wrote a poem on Karma and this, too, I wrote,

> I brushed aside the curtain of the window of mine eyes
> and beheld the sparkling truth that within me did reply,
> 'You're not this house of flesh and bone,
> which sleeps decays and dies.
> You are immortal consciousness,
> Lord of the earth and the skies.'

Fate and Free-Will

> Yesterday's freewill karma
> guides your Fate today.
> Today's freewill karma
> mould your Fate tomorrow.

Our past freewill actions have moulded themselves to guide our present choices as per our past desires. – This is Karma.

It is your choice, your limitation is your choice, for you have limited yourself by your past Karma, which has frozen around you now.

And you have to bear what you did in the past and when you finish that you will be free for future Karma. You see, there is wet mud, which is the present Karma now. In the wet mud you make a nice bed for yourself, and you say I want to sleep at this angle, like this, then after about three or four hours or one or two days the mud dries up then it takes that form which you have made. You have to sleep like this. You want to sleep straight, but you yourself made your mud bed now it is dried up and has limited you. By your past karma you have fashioned the lifestyle of today and now you want to act in a different way? You must first live the lifestyle that you yourself have designed. The bed is now dried up it has to be in this shape, when you have wriggled out of that bed then you can fashion another lifestyle. Once your Karma has frozen into your subconscious mind, you have to bear the consequences of the Karma that you yourself have created. The Karma that you create today, you will live tomorrow. Because they are space time frames, plates in your subconscious mind, so whatever you impress upon your mind today shall come before you tomorrow unless you can go faster than light and change your past. You cannot reverse time because you are slower than light, so for that you have to be faster than light – faster than time. But then you will be playing God, you will be playing the drama of God like Babaji, which would take a long, long time for all of us to do.

What we can do is Kriya Yoga now. The gentle abrasion of whose breath wears away limiting karma and creates freedom Karma.

If you plant all cactus trees in the garden outside and go to Spain, when you come back the next year you will find all cactus plants growing in the garden and then you will cry, "oh, why didn't I get roses? Why did I get cactus? I want a rose plant." Well, you should have planted rose plants last year, then you would have got rose plants this year. So, the Law of Karma is very exact and very just. You get what you deserve, your actions are just a reflection of your past reactions. Therefore, learning this lesson do the correct actions now, whose reactions you will enjoy in the future.

Part V
Yogic Cosmology

Hold Steadfast to Spiritual Practice

Aum Ananda-mAnanda kara Prasannam,
Gnyana Swaroopam Nijabodha Roopam,
Yogendra Midhiyam bhavarogya vaidhyam,
Srimad Gurum nityam aham bhajami. Aum.

When we begin our meditations in Kriya Yoga, there is a set of techniques which are given to us to practice which will unfold the inner being. We always begin our spiritual practice, with the Omkar Kriya, I am now going to give. You must remember that as I speak, my words will penetrate your heart and give you healing transmissions and a spiritual boost. My words will evolve your inner emotional body, mental body and intuitional body. So now, the first technique which we call the Omkar technique is to do with creation and how we reverse the process whereby we have come.

All of you have heard of the Big Bang theory, that at the beginning of creation there was the Word and the Word was with God and God was the Word. That word is Omkar meaning that which glorifies the Lord and Creation. So Omkar itself is chanting God within you. It is a sacred word and the technique is very simple. I will explain to you step by step.

During the Omkar technique, we take a sacred little room to ourselves for a meditation. We face the eastern direction of the rising sun and sit down to meditate. Those who cannot sit down can sit on a chair and insulate their feet with a blanket. And then sit in the aura of love. Whatever the situation, whatever the circumstances, we must hold steadfast to our spiritual practice. We must be constant in our devotion to God, whether it be through Bhajan or Kirtan, which we call spiritual discourse or devotional chanting.

Yogic Science of Creation Explained

Incomprehensible reality spewed out the whole of creation. into cosmic by the sacred Light-sound of Omkar. We need to invoke the sacred sound of creation. We came into creation by the seed sound.

Smaller than the nucleus of an atom, the seed of Omkar lay in the bosom of eternity for eons, for billions of years. And then when the time was ripe, from the Reality was the Great Deep happened creation. the seed sound exploded with an ineffable explosion. It is called the sound of the instant creation, and that sound was Om. In the beginning was the word and the word was with God and God was the word. Therefore, we always start our meditations with the Omkar Kriya. So, with this sound of the instant creation, it explodes from the womb of the Divine Mother called the Great Deep – Amba, Durga, Ambika are the names of the Indian goddesses. The meaning is "she who is unfathomable" – who knows no limits. And God willed it.

The sound of Omkar was the potential in the bosom of the Divine Mother, the Holy Spirit of the universe, which led to tension in the transcendental Matrix. Matrix is a mispronunciation of the Sanskrit word "matrika" or "matrik". The universal matrik is called "Padmamatrika". Padma means "the divine lotus". And the jewel in the lotus is the Omkar, the seed sound. And God was the word – the sound of Om. When He came through creation, He animated the Padmamatri, mother. Do you see people also calling their mother, for short, "ma"? So, "ma" is a very casual word for representing the Divine Mother, coming from the Sanskrit word, "Padmamatri".

The whole universe lay in the homogeneous fabric of silent, Lightless light. Not a ruffle was there. Then the Omkar – the sound of the instant creation exploded with an inconceivable "big bang" – and within a trillionth of a second, she produced a baby as big as the universe. How could she do it? Because she's the Divine Mother – the Relativity of Reality. So, there was hardly any time, and it was almost as big as the present universe. The little bit of the rest of the universe is taking millions and billions of years to expand to its fullest size. This is the state of creation called the expanding Creator, the expanding Brahma.

You know in timeless teachings of India they have Brahma the creator, and the same being becomes Vishnu the preserver, and Shiva the destroyer of materialism – the big crunch – and the regenerator of spiritual knowledge. So now we are expanding with the great primeval seven quasars at the end of the universe, produced almost at the beginning of time. Then the universe will go into a "steady state" – we have in quantum physics the "steady state" theory – and this is the state of Vishnu the preserver. So the universe is preserved in the state of Vishnu. And then after three hundred eleven trillion, hundred and ten billion, four hundred millions and thousands of years, will come the "big crunch", and you go into the super massive, the "Great Beyond Time", the Mahankal. This is Shiva – He About Whom We Know Nothing. You have the Expander, the Pervader, and Redeemer! One About Whom We Know Nothing. And He engulfs everything – time and space are not. Time was not, space was not, and all lay in that bosom of eternity, ineffable and unspeakable, ParamShiva. So that's why, when we try to go back to the source of Shiva and beyond, into the essence of the Great Reality, we practice the reverse technique of His expanding word called Omkar – the sacred word. And when we practice this in our spinal cord, we are expediting the process and evolving ourself into our own parent source, and Divine Consciousness.

Psychological and Chronological Yugas of Time

Can we find enlightenment now or must we wait for the enlightenment of humanity?

The yugas are durations of time. But there are two times. There's the external time, the chronological time, and yugas are for the masses. There's another yuga which is a psychological yuga, which is for the individual. The degree and intensity of your Gravity of Samadhis. Yoga will compress the yugas to how you want it. Even to a second. A whole yuga can pass by in a second. The psychological time can be expedited. The chronological time will remain the same for others, but it matters not, because the person changing the psychological time into zero time can pass through his own stargate into self-realization.

I'll give you an example how to understand this. When I was small, we used to have mathematical lessons and forty-five minutes was the duration of the math class. It appeared like three hours. Then we had another class, painting and arts. That was forty-five minutes and it appeared like ten minutes, fifteen minutes. And then when we were small, in kindergarten, upper and low kindergarten, we had a class called sleeping class in the nursery, where the kids have to sleep for half an hour. That passed in ten minutes, five minutes. So with what you like more, time flies. And time drags on with what you dislike. So it's your mind – the degree of concentration determines the duration of time. If your mind is more concentrated, psychological time will be brief. If your mind is staggered, psychological time will drag on. Chronological time will remain the same unless the chronological master, that is, the great mind of the Creator, decides to concentrate. Then he can make the world disappear in the wink of an eye. Causation, space and time break down. The space-time continuum breaks down because of the intense gravity of concentration. Where there's more gravity applied, it shrinks. So also, the yugas, which are to be determined by you. Your own personal yuga. If you're constantly in bliss and light, dear soul, you are not in Kali Yuga, you are in Satya yuga. And even if Satya yuga comes for the masses and your mind is a hellhole, well dear soul, you're in Kali yuga. So, your individual time, your psychological time can be determined by the intensity of the practice of your Kriya Yoga and the gravity of your Samadhis.

You said death is certain. Why is there so much fear about that? and what happens after death?

Body death is another form of life and you as consciousness are immortal. We love death. Death is fleeting, time waits for no man. So, let's make the most of it – let's realize God in this life. Otherwise, when you die you go through the whole process of limbo, the bardo thodol. Which we call in our tradition devasthanam. We go through the astral sphere – the bhurloka, bhuvarloka, svarloka, maharloka, janaloka, tapoloka, satyaloka. You go through all these loka; then you go to partala, rasatala, talatala, all the various hells for all the bad you've done and all the various heavens for the good you've done. So before this whole rigmarole starts, then you take birth in a human body and come again, where you can start your Kriya Yoga again. So instead of going around all the way when you know death is certain, time is fleeting, let's catch the train. Let's get our passport to paradise done in this life. Stamped and clear. Samadhi is the stamp. Meditation is the stamp. So it's a question of time. We don't want to waste time. We'd like to meet our beloved Lord in this life. In this life. Therefore, with that urgency we're saying because time is fleeting,
>   Let not precious moments slip by.
> Seek now the ultimate truth, oh soul swan,
>   Spread your wings to fly
>   Immortal realms which death defy.

Yogiraj Gurunath Siddhanath

The Rings Pass Not

What are the Rings pass not?

Rings past not are the varying electro-magnetic, mind-fields through which Consciousness passes to expand into Kaivalya, the Singularity. Yes, that's a paradigm shift. That is the wave particle duality, where the particle becomes the wave. The electron becomes light. This is passing the first mandala of the rings pass not. When you connect with the Guru, if you read my Patanjali Sutras book, there are three mandalas that you have to pass. The first mandala of rings pass not where the electron becomes light. The second mandala of the rings pass not where the space time continuum breaks down, where the speed of the light exceeded. That is the second paradigm shift, when the speed of the light is exceeded, you go into a time-reversed phenomenon. The third phase of the rings pass not is when all creation is reversed into its transcendental matrix. And when your consciousness enters that Reality, all, even the finer state I unveiled and you enter the Kaivalya – Pure Incomprehensible Consciousness. When you know that the whole of the creation is a wave motion – it is but relativity – you pass in to the great void. You are passing through the star of what we know not what. In the singularity, when that light and space and time have all been swallowed up, there shines a star of you know not what. This is passing the third mandala. Because if the black hole as you call it, swallows up light, then how can be there a dazzling star in the singularity when it swallowed up light? As I've told it, Babaji is the star of we know not what – he confounds us. He is the dichotomy. He is a visible and invisible saviour of mankind. He is the nameless one, and yet goes by many names. The avatars and the great Gods have not been able to fathom the transcendental star. Do not try to transcend his cosmic transcendental star. It is inconceivable. We know it cannot be done. But for the sake of people, out of compassion, he is here to tell you passing the mandala of the rings of pass not, in His lofty descent to humanity.

The star of 'the know not what' is Babaji. And when light and space and time have all been swallowed up and there is the great nothing and great void and yet the star shines, that is Babaji. When you pass that star, all Avatars become Maha-Avatars. That is also called the land of no returns and that is the finality Kaivalya. Just before that, the stage is the centre everywhere and the circumference nowhere. So these are the three mandalas of rings pass not. One is exceeding the electron – the paradigm shift from the electron to the light. The second one is exceeding the speed of light, going backward in time phenomenon. Passing the third mandala of rings pass not, space and time all disappear into great void and there is no light. Yet a certain star, shines in the darkness which cannot be comprehended. This is the star of we know what not what. This is Babaji. Passing that, the third mandala of rings pass not, is a total and Absolute Enlightenment.

What is the star that we pass in Jyothi Mudra and Shiva Netra Bhedan? Is that the star? One is the individual star and the other is the cosmic star. The individual star is penetrating, the individual star of Savikalpa /Asmita Samadhi is through Divine mind of electron. Penetrating the Cosmic Star of Babaji is of Divine Consciousness and the lightless light, where space-time continuum breaks down. The electron represents the world ego and from these you go into light. It is the electron of asmita or ego samadhi – Savikalpa Samadhi of I-am-ness meaning I pervade creation fabric, - all of this is me. When you penetrate the electron of Savikalph Samadhi, you go into a state of Nirvikalpa Samadhi, and there every individual is enlightened. But is this enlightenment the same as the enlightenment of the great one by the Avatars, passing through the star of Lightless Light Maha-Avatar Babaji in the cosmic sphere and going into the great Is-ness of zero not zero? No! That is absolutely cosmic God realization. This is absolute self-realization, because passing through the star you have crystal mind – you have no karma. The only difference is the residual karmas of your past life, of past world cycles, are still to be worked out in the stage of Nirvikalpa Samadhi and in that stage, Kaivalya, the final one in the cosmic sphere, you pass through the third mandala of rings pass not - the star of we know not what. In that, there is absolutely no residual karma of this or past lives. It is beyond enlightenment - Athi maha parinirvana - The space-time continuum breaks down and he Star of Lightless Light of Babaji which shines in the Singularity is passed or not passed?

> Who art thou I know thee not and yet I am of thee
> We cannot comprehend thee Lord thou Emperor of Divinity
> I sit and melt in silence in Thy Love oh Infinite
> Make me thy truth make me thy Love Eternal Lord of Light!!!

Yogiraj Gurunath Siddhanath

Stages of Samadhi and
Sri Yukteswar's Work at Hiranyalok

I am here to serve humanity as my larger self, and the best way we can serve humanity is to give them the inner knowingness of self-realization. Today, for all the people who are hearing me, I am going to speak something out of my own experience and connected with the work that the Gyan Avatar Sri Yukteswar is doing in a heavenly sphere called Hiranyalok. Now, it is said that every individual human being has a mind field – an individual mind field. You know like you have a magnetic field, you have a mind field also. You have an individual mind field and you have a community mind field – the people who you are connected with in your local community. Then you have a country mind field, and a global mind field. You are also connected to a universal mind field.

The mind field is made up of the substance of all your actions and reactions when you live in the duality of maya – the duality of your day-to-day life. You interact with people and create impressions, thought forms, and remembered samskars – experiences of past lives. As you practice your day-to-day meditation, you clear your physical body, your astral body, your mental body, and your intuitional body. The physical body has more limited mind field. The astral body has bigger, emotional one. Then the mental body has a bigger mind field, and your causal body is spread over the universe. The universal causal body has a universal mind field.

And as you practice meditation, you first get into the process of dharana, which is concentration. Focusing your mind on the object which you would like to pay attention to is called concentration. Then you further go, after concentrating, to a state called meditation. In meditation, you clear your thoughts. Superfluous thoughts of your mind, which is fidgety and chattering all the while, are cleared. After dharana to you go to dhyana. Concentration, meditation and ecstasy, are dharana, dhyana, and samadhi. You go to the first stage of samadhi after meditation.

When you focus your mind on an object, your mind distracts from the object of your attention. You have to pull it back again and again and apply it to that object. Say you are focussing on a flame – you try to look at a flame, and after some time a bang goes or somebody calls and you get distracted. Again you bring your attention back to the flame. So that practice of bringing your mind again and again to the focus of your attention is called the practice of concentration. The moment that practice is perfected, it no longer remains concentration. That perfected concentration is meditation or dhyana, where uninterrupted and steadily, you go into a phase of focused awareness. The object is still gross. Then in samadhi you are still in a subtler mind state – you go from the gross element to subtler attributes of the flame like heat, the orange color, the spiritual significance of light and the flame. All these things happen in samadhi, which is called ecstasy.

It is said that people who are practising and doing Kriya Yoga and meditation, through long years of practise, cleanse their minds to a great degree. I have experienced in my meditation that the mind has three basic layers. The first and superfluous layer which can be cleared in meditation is called thoughts, which are known as vritti. Vritti means thoughts or fluctuations of the mind. These thoughts by regular practice can be disciplined and brought under control by concentration and meditation. Then you get to a deeper layer of the mind. For that, you have to go into a deeper level which is called samadhi. You become partially integrated with the object of your concentration. The integration is called focused awareness. Suppose you are focusing on an apple, you partially tend to partake of the apple. Then as you go into a deeper samadhi, where you go internal, the gross association with the apple melts away and you totally become one with the apple. Your awareness is totally focused on the entirety of the apple. A deeper state of samadhi would be where the form of the apple begins to melt and you are focused only on the sweetness of the apple, the shape of the apple, redness of the color. The grosser form melts and only the attributes of the apple you are absorbed in remain. But this is all in a state of mind.

When your mind is cleared of all its thoughts, you go into the final state of the mind awareness, into the universal field of mind where all your thoughts have disappeared, and you go deeper into that last state of samadhi. You have not entered divine consciousness, but you are still in the state of divine mind, which in technical language we call Savikalpa Samadhi or Samprajnata Samadhi – the samadhi with prajnat, with cognition, with perception, and with knowledge. In this last stage of samadhi, you also get rid of the deeper thought forms – experiences which have happened previously. This deepest layer of the mind is called 'samskars' or remembered experiences

– impressions in the deep collective subconscious. And yet deeper than this third stage of remembered experiences are remembered experiences of past lives. When you get rid of all these experiences, then and then alone can you attain enlightenment.

Now let us go the stage of Savikalpa Samadhi, the final layer, which we also call Samprajnata Samadhi, where your awareness expands to the size of the cosmos. You can feel and know yourself as being present everywhere. It is a very high state of expanded divine mind. When you go to the state of expanded divine mind, you have already finished with the fluctuations of your mind. The first layer of your mind is clear. The second layer is also clear, and it becomes a homogeneous fabric of one thought. Let's say feeling of I am-ness Asmit Samadhi – I am Brahma; I am divine; I am the universal mind field. So, your mind becomes one homogeneous fabric of tranquil lake – one electron. But you are still in the state of divine mind. This is the state of Savikalpa Samadhi – Samprajnata Samadhi.

To enter to the state of Asamprajnata Samadhi, which is Nirvikalpa Samadhi, you have to transit from the stage of divine mind of Samprajnata Samadhi. You are transiting from divine mind to divine consciousness. Every time you transit, anybody transits, he has to pass through the pure state of mind called the Bindu, which we in Kriya Yoga and Patanjali Yoga call the Transcendental Star – the Kutastha Chaithanya or the permanent state.

I always tell people, follow the way of the purple star of the East, which ultimately purifies and becomes white or colourless. When you penetrate from divine mind, it becomes the divine consciousness. Of course, the star is representing trinity in duality – the golden rim of the third eye of the star. The third eye is the golden rim pale, but intense golden light. It is the holy spirit of Brahma. The blue centre represents the Krishna consciousness, the Christ Consciousness Vishnu, and the scintillating white star, the purple, white star in the centre represents the God Father Shiva in duality and relativity.

Once you penetrate the star, you go from divine mind of relativity into divine consciousness of singularity. Beyond this state, there is a place called Hiranyalok where Sri Yukteswar trains people to go from Nirvikalpa Samadhi to higher and more permanent states of Nirvikalpa Samadhi. After all, Nirvikalpa Samadhi is the very pure state of divine consciousness, in which you have no Karma, no thoughts, no whirlpools of mind fluctuations, no thought ideas,

The Reality of Kriya Yoga

no experiences, and no samskars also. But in that state, you still cannot get to further states of Nirvikalpa Samadhi or Asamprajnata Samadhi. The further state is called Nirbija Samadhi, or Seedless Samadhi, where remembered experiences of past lives are also there. These experiences may be from a hundred years ago, a past lifetime, or a past world cycle, but if you carry that thought impression in your universal mind field, you cannot be enlightened perfectly like Buddha was enlightened or the Krishna was enlightened. Of course, Maha Avatar Babaji we do no know – that's way beyond that Enlightenment of any Avatar or immortal. Sri Yukteswar is enlightened or Lahiri Mahaysaya is enlightened. They were Gyan Avatar and Yoga Avatar respectively.

I often give certain states of thought-free awareness, the Nirvichara Samadhi. When I give these states, all the thoughts of people, the audience disappear. The vritti – the thought forms or ideas – disappear. But the past life samskars or the samskars which have been previously done are not necessarily wiped out. That has to be done in deeper samadhi, the Nirbeej Samadhi. I am able to exhibit this only because of the grace of Babaji. His divine grace allows me to transfer this state of no-mind – a thought-free state of pure awareness to everyone who listens to me and who hears my talks. Even now as I am talking to you, you will find yourself thought-free, because I have no mind. I have an awareness, given by the Lord God Babaji – Shiva-Goraksha-Babaji. This is the tool I use to serve humanity as my larger self with all your blessings and good wishes.

When Sri Yukteswar works, he takes these people to a thought-free pure awareness called the Nirvikalph Samadhi or the Asamprajnata Samadhi. He is sharing the universal soul consciousness. The divine mind has been put away, as you have passed through the star from the third dimension to fourth, fifth and sixth dimensions. When Sri Yukteswar works, when you go in to the state of pure awareness, you have to segregate your pure consciousness, even if it will be for the time being, from remembered experiences of your past life, which are the residual impressions of your mind. But you'll ask me, how does the mind enter the star? Even entering the star, remembered experiences of past lives are not done with. You as a soul consciousness transit, your consciousness transits, from divine mind to divine consciousness. So, the conscious here transits. But remembered experiences of past lives are not in your soul consciousness when you transit from the third dimension to higher dimensions – from the duality to the singularity and from the relativity of the divine mind to the reality of divine consciousness. But these remembered experiences of past lives, which are not in your consciousness, but are residual of past life experiences, have to be worked out. They lie as dormant Karma and are called out to be neutralized. Just to work that out, your consciousness has to come again and again into the mind's lake to work out that remembered experiences of the past life till each and every thought, each and every shred, each and every molecule and atom of that past life karma has been worked out. So it's not an easy job. Sri Yukteswar is in a very high place to do this.

You see, a long time back, Gautam Buddha was walking the plains of this earth. The light of the world, Lord Buddha. He was the first one to make the effort from being a normal human being to be one with the gods and be totally enlightened in this world cycle. In former world cycles there were Buddhas. There was Vasishta; there was Brigu; there was Agastya; there was Parashara. There were great and mighty beings, but in this life, it was Siddhartha. Vyasa was the highest of Masters, when he appeared to write Mahabharata with Lord Krishna, who was the Divine Avatar and did not evolve from human – he always was with the divine essence. But Veda Vyasa later incarnated as Gautama Buddha, and he attained enlightenment. They are one and the same person – Veda Vyasa and Gautama Buddha.

So, Sri Yukteswar is in Hiranyalok, transforming people, from Nirvikalpa to higher seedless-Nirbija – from enlightenment to go to further enlightenment, whatever the name may be. And you cannot pass through the final samadhi unless you get to this stage. Of course, Lahiri Mahasaya is also working in higher stages.

So, this is a very interesting thing, and you have to work on how will you segregate it. You will segregate it by always disconnecting your Atma from Buddhi like in paravasta. At lower states also and starve the mind so that it dissolves. But the mind does not stop itself – it does not disappear, even in samadhi. It is the feeling of I-am-ness of the Universe (the veil of the cosmic ego). This Great Illusion of I-am-ness with the samskars are removed only in the final stage of Dharma Megh Samadhi You even have to renounce the desire for the God. You have to renounce the desire for knowledge. First, there is information, then there is intuitional knowledge, then there is divine knowledge and beyond divine knowledge, that is omniscience – Pure Awareness. We do not know what it is. It is the supreme Reality, and this is the stage and great work of Sri Yukteswar, the Gyan Avatar, and Lahiri Mahasaya, the Yoga Avatar.

After those great works, you enter into what is called the Dharma Megha Samadhi, the cloud of virtues. Dharma Megha Samadhi is not a material cloud or form. It is the cloud of virtues when you pass through the very gunas, The Universal Mind-field. Then the great inward turning takes place and you enter into the ineffable, nonpareil, indescribable light of the final, Maha Pari Nirvana – the 'Final Kaivalya' – with your centre everywhere and your circumference nowhere. The Lord of the Irradiant Splendour shines in his own glory with nothing to compare with, nothing to talk about, nothing to say with. That's right, nobody is been able to describe this state. I am just describing it in feeble words to give you an idea – a faint dream idea. My word has darkness, as the dark night, and words irradiant splendour are darkness compared to the real irradiant splendour of the reality of Kaivalya – the Naked Singularity.

Gautama Buddha went to a similar person when he was practising. He got through the stages very fast and went to two teachers: Aaradhya Kalam and Udraka Ramaputra. They pronounce it differently in English texts, but Ramaputra was such a yogi that he was enlightened and an avatar Vibuthi. He never gave initiation on the physical plane – he will always give it at Hiranyalok, the super astral plane. So when Gautama Buddha went and sat before him, he wouldn't talk. Buddha wanted Ramaputra to accept him as his disciple. So, Buddha went into meditation with him face-to-face and he attained to that state where the Guru appeared astrally before him like Sri Yukteswar would appear in Hiranyalok. I've been giving you the parallel, because you people say how fortunate Gautama was. He was, but you have people here who are great rishis and munis, vibuthis and avatars also. Eyes and ears see not. Open your eyes and see. So he went there and then Ramputra initiated him in the astral plane, in the divine Hiranyalok. But Gautama Buddha even that very lifetime passed beyond that state also and then that master said, "I've finished my work, now you have to go to the higher." Then that was the greatness of the Siddharth, the Sakyamuni, that he did it on his own. The first human being in this world cycle to break the sound and light barrier to pass the rings pass not. Then, of course, you have these great Buddhas and this is the parallel case, which I wanted to tell you about. The more you hear of this, the more you absorb it. But people do not know this and are misguided by super marketers of yoga and techniques in the east, north, south, and west.

You have to get to the proper Master. How you can get to that is by sincerely praying to your own inner Guru, the divine in-dweller. O Lord! Please take me to the true Master! And he will do the rest.

Om Nama Shivaya!

The Cosmic Mind is Hiranya Garbha

The cosmic mind is Hiranya Garbha. It would come to that. Ultimately, the Hiranya Garbha is a transcendental matrix. Garbha means the womb; Garbha means matrix. In America. they produce pictures called Matrix and all, but when you ask them what the matrix is, they do not know. It comes from the word matrica – the cosmic mother. And in the medieval ages, during the time of inquisition, the Christian, Catholic and then the Islamic movements did all they could to suppress feminine principle in nature. No female! Forget the feminine principle, forget the womb, forget the feminine organs. They are taboo.

You know this – I am repeating the history. If you read history, there were nuns who were working for humanity and serving and the men came and shut it down and they did their own rituals and functions. This was a partial process of evolution, where the male hormones try to dominate the feminine principle and wipe out all that is feminine. Father, Son and the Holy Ghost. No! No! It's too feminine. India clearly says Father, Mother, Son. How can it be without the other counterpart? The living proof of the existence of women is in front of us here – why have they made them disappear? How can you make them disappear when you yourself are born from the woman? How foolish was the medieval man – that was the age of very, very ugly machoism. But there was a noble quality of chauvinism in machoism. Chauvinistic people did not vote for this or did not think that it is right, but the machoistic quality in the chauvinist destroyed the feminine principle, and this is very, very wrong. The feminine principle, the mother aspect, has to be given its place, so therefore I am teaching the truth. It is not whether I like it or not - it is a fact. Therefore, the transcendental matrix is the Hiranya Garbha. Garbha is the matrix. In every Church, when you go to the left-hand side is a vestry. Gurunath has said in his poetry. The Mystic wine, the bishop's wine, says

The Reality of Kriya Yoga

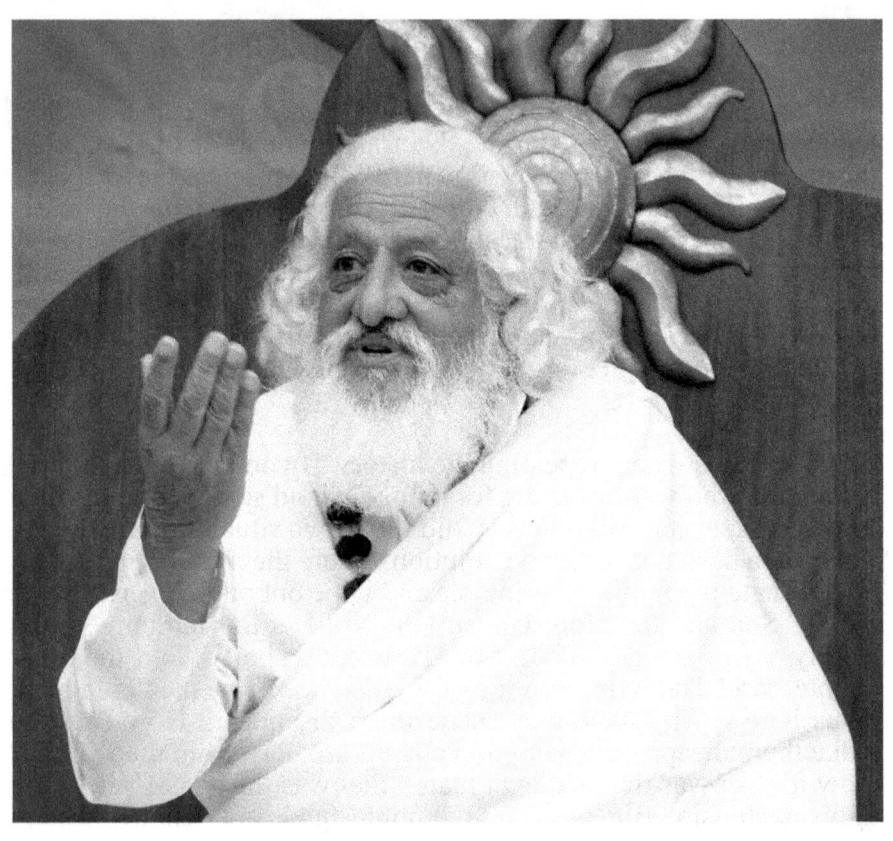

Yogiraj Gurunath Siddhanath

Time spent in solitude
"In the vermilion vestry of his mind,
grew exotic grapes of rarest kind.
Where silence stills the finest brew,
that wine it tastes like honey dew"

Part VI
Yoga and the West

The Reality of Kriya Yoga

Vegetarianism and Meditation

You see, it's been a great source of concern to me that people are consuming tomatoes and lettuce with great voracity. And the tomatoes and lettuces have a nervous system. This is most worrying to me, and the Indian Scientist Jagadish Chandra Bose also discovered that they had feelings. Now, we must stop this, Herbivorism is a crying shame.

How can you harm a poor tomato? Or an orange or tangerine? And an apple – ruthlessly digging your teeth into the apple. To top it off, you skin the apple. I asked them why do you skin it? They said pesticides. But pesticides is not my concern; the apple is my concern. The tomato is my concern. May I ask you, what are we doing in this direction of preventing the eating of lettuce and tomatoes and the green chilis and all the vegetarian food? If they only had a nervous system, okay, I can let it go. But they have emotions? Basic emotions? Has anyone thought of this ever before? Those Vegans that are playing holier than thou and talking about cruelty to animals ought to be ashramed of themselves. It's vegetable carnage.

If you're a vegetarian, should you be a vegetarian? Should you eat meat? Does it matter as long as you do your kriya?

I think that it does matter as far as cruelty and all this is concerned. It also matters because meat and beef is very heavy and makes you a numbskull. Especially the beef. We avoid it because it's very thick, it has a lot of uric acid, so it makes the brain thick. It's not meant for meditation. It also has a lot of adrenaline, which comes into the meat, because before the animal is led to slaughter, it emits a hormone of fear through the adrenaline flight mechanism. This hormone is eaten by us day in and day out, so we also get the fear complex. Therefore, meat should totally be avoided.

I have fasted on liquids and all that for two or three months. But I'm going to try to clear the thing: I'm not saying you should eat meat and I'm not saying you should not eat meat. I'm not saying you should eat lettuce; I'm not saying you should not eat tomatoes. I'm not saying anything. I'm just trying to get your mind straight – that any material thing, whether it be fish, beef, goat, lamb, tomatoes, lettuce, is made up of electron, protons, and neutrons. It's a material thing that is in relativity. And therefore, it's just a part of the food chain for all men and animals. You individually must decide what you have to eat - whether to live on celery, or whether you want to have turkey breast, or whether you want to have chicken, whether you want to have pastas and tofu and salads. It's all up to you. This is the food chain. You have to get on with your Kriya Yoga – that's the first point. Now, in the food chain, what is good? I would say vegetarianism, because meat is not conducive to meditation. Finished. That's it. Above all Realize that all beings are the Immortal Soul and not the corruptible body and there the problem of diet is solved. Its all the food chain because the Soul can never die!

The Self
From Burning Man to Rainbow Man

Speaking of gurukul system, we have done a wonderful thing here in America. We've not only formed a group of like-minded people, but we have actually formed a gurukul system. This is like a gurukul because the same people are constantly coming again and again and the same people are developing very steadily, and we are able to hold a lot of our people. In spite of them going to Burning Man, they still come back here. They go to Disneyland or reggae on the river or Burning Man – that's their life. That's the maverick and revolutionary style of a new evolving spirit: the free spirit in human beings.

But they always come back to something which is of the source and ancient traditions and systems, because of the experience which they got here, which they cannot get there. They are finding out that the real peace that they're seeking is not exactly there, but here. They're finding that the other peace is coming to them like an avalanche from without, while the peace that's given here is coming from within. So, they say: "that's very interesting. My rational mind is saying 'go to Burning Man.', but my intuitional mind is saying 'go to Gurunath'." The reason for this is that the rational mind desires the normal way of thinking and having fun, but the true fun is in the inner quiet of the mind. And as they mature into this by their practise, as they grow into this, they find that it is better to be steady within. Not that they should leave those entertainment venues. Of course not. But they should never leave this tranquillity. So, it's important to know that the answer lies within.

You've got to burn from within out. Not outwards in. You put your hand in fire, you'll get singed. But if the fire is your very own nature, and if it comes from the nectar of your Soul, then it shall not burn you. Because it knows you. You are friends. It's the inner fire of Kundalini. The Burning Man you're looking for is within you. It is the Kundalini Fire, which comes from within and goes without. That is the Burning Man. That's the true meaning of the Burning Man.

What does the fire burn? It burns your lust, your greed, your passion, your attachments, and the frivolousness of your mind. And in its burning, in its burning for Babaji, in its burning for honesty, it gives you faith, integrity, and courage. So, these qualities are gained by self-effort. The answer lies within. And if you can burn from within without, you shall be transformed into the Rainbow Man. And you shall be the king of the rainbow gatherings. So lose not hope. You shall be the Rainbow Man with lightning speed. From Burning Man to Rainbow Man, that's the beauty of the Kundalini, It transforms you into the Rainbow Man of light and love and truth and power and wisdom.

The Benefits of Awakening Kundalini with the Science of Kriya Yoga

I've heard that people shake their bodies – is that related to Yoga or meditation?

Shakers and Movers. The Quakers. The Quakers, the Amish, and the Shakers and the Movers. When they had their body shaking, there was no science to contain it, so they didn't know what was happening to them. The Quakers used to quake; the Shakers used to shake. And the Wakers, when they reached their state, used to wake.

About the shaking, this is the kundalini. Those people who don't do Mahamudra, they shake because the toxins are being thrown out of their body and their body quivers. Then they shake and perspire and speak in many tongues. And they shall speak in many tongues, people from all over. Then Jesus, the Christ, came. When he went into the crowds, his radiance automatically catharted them. And when they threw out the negativity of their karma, they quaked and they shaked and they moved, and they became purified by that process during those times.

We have developed the science of Kriya Yoga – Mahamudra – which would channelize the energy of kundalini in your spine and emote through the exhalation of your breath, burning your negativity. So there will be no shaking and quaking and you will get to a higher level of consciousness without creating an undue emotional upheaval in your system. But sometimes during this path, there is an identity crisis – there's an emotional crisis. When you go towards God, you feel scared, you feel frightened, you feel you are losing your identity. These things are reduced. They will be there, but they are mitigated by the scientific path of yoga and meditation that you are following.

God is Everywhere, So Why Meditate?

God is everywhere. Many companies are saying "God is everywhere; we love God," but they are raiding – they are making a fraud of billions of dollars. So I know God is everywhere and you know God is everywhere. And so what? The world is carrying on fudging and cheating and 'gooding' and loving.

It's you and I who have to change, the world will not change for us. God is everywhere, but you and I do not realize God. If we realized God in this world, if humanity was a realized humanity, there would be no murders, no killings, and no invasions and taking over countries. The Muslim knows that God is everywhere – that Allah is everywhere – and the Christians also know and the Catholics know that God is everywhere. And they're shooting and killing one another and raiding one another's countries. And God is everywhere.

It's good God is everywhere, but how does that affect you and me? Just by saying God is everywhere, he does not become everywhere. God is in you also, but Kriya Yoga asks you the question: Are you in God? No, you are not in God. For God to be in you and you to realize God within you, you must practice Kriya Yoga and evolve to the Realization.

It's very easy to say: since God is everywhere, I am God, so let me have my whiskey and my cigarettes, and let me consort, and dance on Fiji Island. There are people like that, but they are deceiving themselves. They are lazy, self-deceptive people, who do not want to face the realities of the world, nor make the spiritual effort to realize the Divine In-dweller.

Merely talking philosophy does not make you God-Realized. You must take the first step to God, then He will take ten steps towards you. But you can't just sit and say God is everywhere. Philosophy must be backed by reality. Christ said, "I am one with God." He told Lazarus, "Lazarus, take up thy bed and walk. Wake." He raised the dead. If these parrot philosophers also go and say, "hey, dead man, rise!" Will the dead man rise? Christ was reality who spoke philosophy. The other philosophers are an empty bubble who cannot do what they talk.

At the marriage at Canaan, Christ said, "okay, now the water will be changed to wine." The philosopher will also say, "by the mutation of atoms we can change the water to wine." But when you ask him to change the water to wine, he cannot do it. So, a person who has no reality, no realization, cannot afford to speak philosophy.

Virtue, Sin, and Guilt

Let us not be discouraged if you get thoughts of depression, lust, or greed or aggression during your meditations. That's the natural you who has been practising aggression, practising lust. Why shouldn't a person enjoy what he most easily enjoys? The thing he most easily enjoys is obviously sex. So, there's no big deal about that, because you are behind the ecstasy of sex. They call it orgasm, but actually it's a spark of Divine Ecstasy. It gives you that feeling, and for one second when you finish you go into a state of blank when there is no thought. Everybody goes into no-mind. That's the time you contact your soul. And we're not talking about morality, we're talking about Truth. I'm cutting the agency and the trappings of all religion and hypocrisy. I'm getting to the core, I'm talking about Truth. That is the time that each one of you has experienced that tremendous peace after the act of uniting with your partner. That perfect peace – the No-Mind. That is the soul contact. I am giving you that soul contact on a much subtler and higher level. Where you have no thought, you're living in soul consciousness. And I cannot say I'm giving you my soul consciousness, because at the level of the Universal Soul Consciousness, humanity is One.

Lord Krishna says in the Bhagavad Gita:

> The Atma and the Soul is immortal and Divine.
> The Fire cannot burn it,
> The water cannot wet it
> The breeze cannot dry it
> Weapons cannot pierce it.
> You are pure from moment to moment.
> Forget the past, it is dead and gone.
> From moment to moment I am born anew.
> In every breath, I am pure.
> In every breath, I am born anew.

One galaxy, which is smaller than an atom in God's body, is a hundred thousand light-years across. The rate at which light travels at 300,000 kilometers per second, and if it travels for a hundred thousand years, that is the expanse of the galaxy, which is smaller than an atom in God's body. And then a little boy goes and he pees in his mother's lap. A one-year-old boy, and he says "O, I have sinned! And my mother's clothes have got wet. What shall we do?" The mother doesn't mind, she just changes the nappies if he poops. That's like us asking if we've sinned.

In your hay days you've sowed your wild oats and been a rowdy brat! FORGET IT. These are very, very, very trivial things. Forget Vice and forget Virtue. Make an ash heap of them. Start anew this moment. Every moment is Divine. You are like the Light; you cannot be tainted by good or bad because you are the Truth. The Light is not tainted by me cursing it. Nor purified by me chanting 'Om.' The Light is the Light. The Light is not tainted by me reading a sex book. The Light is not purified by me reading the Bible. But if I put off the Light, I can neither read the Bible nor the sex book. So, the Atma, the Soul, the Divine Holy Spirit in you is like the Light. So have courage. This is where the guilt and fear syndrome should be totally wiped out. The guilt is more of a sin than the so called sin. So, snap out of the guilt and meditate the Flame of purity, see God in it!

The act of sex is not a sin. But the guilt that follows it is a sin. You should have no guilt, otherwise don't do it. So, these are things on which we have no time to waste. If there are people, if there's one thing, I could just pull out of their head is the guilt syndrome and say, "Okay son, carry on. Blaze ahead. You're Divine."

A little boy went, and he peed in the Ocean and said, "ahhh," and then he tasted the water and said, "Salty! Because of me, the Ocean has become salty!" and he flexes his little muscles, this two-year-old boy. And that's like telling the Divine Mother, O Mother, I've peed on your dress. This is how we are. Who the hell are we, trying to tell that this is evil, and this is not?

What strength does this evil have anyway, compared to the vast cosmic scenario? I've told you the width and length of one galaxy which is smaller than an atom. Who the hell are we in that? Are we even nothing?

And then because you both have something, you feel in your little syndrome, your ego, you've committed a sin or a vice or a virtue. God didn't come and say that. Some stupid priests put this syndrome in our head. Some damn psychological thing has gotten stuck in our chromosomes and genes, tampered our DNA in the wrong way and we feel for every little thing we do we are sinners. Totally wrong. It's a wrong teaching – a wrong education. The education of guilt and sin and damnation. I'm sorry it's taught by the Church, but it's very, very wrong.

And we have this generation here that's suffering because of this guilt! This is NOT education! Education is strength! and Truth! and Light! You cannot sin! Vice and Virtue is relative.

This is how I make up this big joke "How can I eat a plant? How can I eat a cabbage which has an emotion?" That's the food chain. You're not the cabbage, neither are you the venison, the deer, nor the lamb. Eat what you like. But don't have a mistaken identity that you are the body and not the soul. You are the soul.

If your soul is of the nature of the Lightless Light, can it be tainted by anyone spitting on it? Have you ever tried to spit on the afternoon Sun? You spit at the Sun, it comes right in your eye. So, you cannot sin. The True You is the Divine Indweller (The Atma).

So have no guilt, have no fear, be soldiers of Light, and march on!

Kriya and the Guilt-Fear Complex

How do we overcome when we think in our past-lives we may have done something evil?

The guilt syndromes – or depression, aggression, or anxiety – these are minor things. When you do the Shiva-Shakti, when you do 144 every day, those aggressions are funnelled into the washing machine of your spinal chord and they come out clean. They are lengthened, washed, and then transformed into light. The transfiguration takes place.

Did you know that the practice of Shiva-Shakti which you are doing is a process of Transfiguration? Did you know that you are being transfigured every time you do it? But you're doing so little that you're being changed very little. You do five hundred every day and in 3 months see what a transfiguration takes place. You won't be able to recognize yourself. This is what Jesus meant by transforming your weaknesses – the darkness, the negativity – into Light, Power, and Truth.

Take control of your life. And practice this – the practice of transfiguration.

There is no Sin. There is no Vice. There is no Virtue. These are all small facets or idiosyncrasies. Of course, if you dwell on a vice, or a guilt-syndrome, and let it make a home in your mind, it would be very damaging. Therefore, we have a meditation called the Pratipaksha Bhavana- meditation. The meditation of opposites. He who feels guilty should feel they are pure and strong. See, there is no such thing as a sin in this world. The only sin is the feeling of guilt that follows the action which is labelled by society as a vice or a virtue.

You take up a gun, you shoot a man, and society says you're a murderer and you get guilt. You take up a gun, you shoot a hundred men with the same gun and society says you're a war hero and you feel great. You get the congressional order of merit. I mean, what the hell is this? Same gun. Same society. Are they trying to make a fool of us?
This is stupid! There is no vice nor virtue. It's the spirit in which it

is done. If you kill for motives which are selfish, they call it a vice. If you kill in honour of saving the country from being run over by another country, it's patriotism. But the gun is the same, the bullets are the same. The life is gone all the same. The one or the hundred who die don't care, they in any case go and evolve. It is you who are stuck with this sin or vice or virtue. What the hell are you wasting your time about? Make an ash heap of vice and virtue! Seek the truth! That's what I say.

You have good karma, and you have bad karma. You have good and you have evil. These are all things which are relative, which are in Maya. The Yogi makes an ash heap of both and seeks directly the truth – O Lord, for You and You alone. And on the Path, as people come by him, he touches them, blesses them, serves them, and assists them along the Path to reach the Final Goal which is the actualization of the essence of their beings.

So this sin, this vice and virtue has been created by the clergy, the ecclesiastical order to leech off and fleece of money from an innocent society who has not a notion about what has happened. Because if there is one boy, and he goes out with a girl, but while going out with the girl, another girl comes and he goes out with the other girl, he feels very guilty that he's cheated out on the first girl. So then, he has to go to church and profess to the priest in the window what his guilt fear and what his sin is or vice is. And that Priest is going out with both the girls. So this is the syndrome – this is how the world goes on. So it's a lovely game. Forget these silly games and just seek the Truth.

> Night and Day O Lord, I burn for thee.
> Whether my wife loves me, I'm happy.
> Whether she hates me, I'm happy.
>
> Success and failure,
> Name and fame,
> To me, a mere dolls' wedding game.
> In joy and sorrow,
> Light and dark,
> I ever that eternal spark!
>
> In honour and dishonour, too,
> The constant Yogi, ever new.

Play the game of the world as it is, but be unaffected by it, just as a lotus on the waters lying, unwetted and undying. In passion, it's not wetted by the waters. It's lying in the waters of Samsara, in the razzmatazz of life. It is in society, but yet, not of society. It is not wetted by the waters of society. Be as a lotus lying – unwetted yet undying. It's not tainted by society, yet it's in society. Be like the light. If you tell the light "OMMM," the light will still be the light. It's not purified by it. Or you say some good things – "oh beautiful Light, how beautiful you are – with your rays you shine upon me. Thank you very much. I am thy humble friend and servant." Nothing will happen to the light. You tell the light, "Damn you." The light is not going to get tainted.

You read, "O Lord, thou art my beloved Heart and Soul. I breathe thy breath – and yea, though I walk through the valley of the shadow of Death, I shall fear no evil, O Lord, for thou art with me. My cup shall be full and I shall follow thee all the days of my Life. Amen, Amen, Amen. In the name of the Father, the Son, and the Holy Ghost. The Pure Holy Ghost." You'll read this, okay? You read the Bible. The light has not been affected by the Bible. You pick up another book. "...as he put his arms around her, he felt his strong grip and she felt a warm glow rushing through her body as he embraced her in his manly arm." And so this is something to do with a very beautiful emotion of man and woman and all. The light is still not affected by it.

Another guy comes and says, "okay, where are the passports?" He says "okay, fudge it" he cheats the signature, he's forging passports. Another fellow is writing a false check. It's all because of the light. The light is not purified or tainted by the actions of the people who do it here, but if you put off the lights none of these things can be done. That is the nature of your soul. That is the nature of God. That is the nature of Atma. It is neither tainted by the bad nor purified by the good. But the light is the light. But if the light is not, neither can you do the bad nor the good. So you are the light. Have no guilt, have no fear. Because you cannot have guilt. There is no vice nor virtue. You, the light, your soul is not tainted by the actions of your emotions, or your mental body or your emotional body. But if the light is not, neither can you forge a check nor read the Bible.

The Atma, the Divine Spirit, is above vice and virtue; good and evil. You are the light. The Divine Light that fills in the chamber of the Hamsa Swan in the Cave of Brahma is your Divine Soul. So have no fear nor guilt. This is what must be taught to children today who are suffering under guilt, anxiety, and aggression. There is no sin! The sin itself is not a sin, but the guilt that follows it is a sin. First wash away the guilt. You are pure from moment to moment. Arise, O soldiers of the Divine, and race to your home sublime.

So, we must teach children purity and confidence and not tell them, "You've sinned, you've done this," already messing up the stuff. So don't do that. Give them courage, give them Light. And explain to them that the Atma is immortal and cannot be affected by your stupid virtue and your vice. Reality is beyond your morality

If you meditate and get on to the clear light, leave these things be. This is not your work. This is not the work of a Hamsacharya to tell children. This is not what we are focused about, are we? We are focused about Kriya Yoga and Hamsa Yoga and teaching the Spiritual Knowledge and Healing.

But I run into family and friends, and I want to do everything I can to help, but I don't know if I'm doing the right thing.

Well, you can help by giving them the Path of God. Give them Kriya Yoga. Give them the Earth Peace meditations. And give them courage. That's all you can give them. You can't give them your soul – you cannot take on their karmas. You're not a superman like Sri Yukteswar, or Babaji, or Ramakrishna or Jesus. You cannot take on the sins of humanity – it needs a superman for that. And we cannot tamper with the karmic law more than what is necessary. We cannot tamper with their DNA. Don't force but lay before them the virtues and benefits of meditation and Kriya Yoga.

Is it an ego trip thinking that I can cure and heal others?

It is an ego trip. If you're getting really deep into this, it's definitely an ego trip. That you think you can cure AIDS, that you can do anything in the world. And, why not? Man has an ego, and the ego will trip. Some days it will trip so bad that it won't get up again. When you heal another your "Prana" does it, and the "I" spoils it.

Now, let's say you know a person being abused. Do you say, "it's karma that needs to be worked out" and let it be? Or do you try

to do something about it?

We should try to help the person as much as we can. Karma will any case take its course, but we go out and help them. We set them on track. We do our best.

Be guilt-free whether you help a person or not. This is karma, let me tell you. This class is strictly spiritual. We are going upon the Path. This is a bifurcation. The karmic law will take care of this. Every action has an equal and opposite reaction. This man will bear the consequences his vice or virtue, because the law of karma is cold and exact. This guy will have to pay for it even if a well-meaning person helps him.

So, be steady. Let's take a cool mind about this. We're all mature people. I really do not know what they mean by vice and virtue. I think this is a very, very relative term concerned firstly with each individual. I would meditate break the bondage of both vice and virtue, karma and be free to be in the infinite Bliss!

But from what you're saying there's still right and wrong? Because you talk about Justice –

Right and Wrong are words in Relativity where "One man's food is another man's poison". So, justice differs for Countries, people and things. They're relative. I could say this is "Bong" and this is "Tong". The Yogi does not mess up his mind or waste time in these arguments, He just sits, goes straight into Samadhi and makes an ash heap of both to get to the final Liberation.

The Truth is that which is experienced. Even that is a relative truth, but if the Yogi says he breathes through you, he must. If he says he'll give you no-mind, he must. A person who walks his talk is closer to the Truth, than the intellectual gymnast, the Sophist wordsmith, or playing the Semantic garnets to convince another.

And if everything is based on the standard of Light, it's not even a fraction of a second in the trammels of the whole universe. It'll take billions and billions of years for light to cover the whole universe. It may never do it. It may change. For me personally, I speak for myself I do not waste time in this vice and virtue phenomena. I give people strength and courage. I say forget the past. Get on the track.

Transcend relativity and get to Reality.

So, first practice the sadhana – that's important. Those people will come to you. The Good Lord will send them to the appropriate people. Your spiritual magnetism will attract the proper people to you. They come because you attract such people. You attract the people you deserve.

Invest in the Everlasting

As the great saint Tukaram has sung, "Oh Lord, let thy thoughts be ever in my mind. Let thy figure, let thy image be ever in my mind, and thy name be ever on my lips." It's a very simple song. When I was small, a yogi and another chap used to come by the back of my house in Pune. There was a small lane. The chap was selling sugar-coated ginger candies. You get them in America now, but they were very tasty. And the yogi used to sing, "If you can't make it now, you will never make it again." I think as a child he was waking me up, you know, to my mission. I felt that I had this burning sensation to run away to the Himalayas. I've written it in my book, Wings to Freedom, how I ran away from home and, after some time, I meditated under a tree and would open one eye to see that whether anybody was looking at me. Nobody looked at me, so I gave it up as a bad joke. And then after three miles I got very tired and then I started to think of the tigers and panthers in the Himalayas.

My uncle and I were running away, but we gave up and went back home. My grandfather didn't even look up from his newspaper – he just carried on. Because he was the boss of the whole territory, and he had his people all over. He knew that the kids would not get lost. So, my first attempted flight into the Himalayas was an utter failure. Later, of course, I was able to go by God's grace. And then the yogi sings, "what are you looking for? When the soul swan leaves the garment of this body and takes flight, or when the soul swan flies, away from this heart, the body will fall like a sack of potatoes and all your wealth will lie waste before you. Oh soul, wake up to your reality. This is not the real wealth. God is the true wealth. All your wealth will be of no use. It will lie waste before you, when the wild goose flies out of your heart." So if you can't make it now, you will never make it then. There's no then, that and the other. It's either now or never. You know? So that's how they tell us. Their way of telling us "Invest in the Everlasting. This evanescent world is but a waking dream.

In the West, they have a now or never different song. They say, "It's now or never, come hold me tight." You know, isn't there a song? So, they are also urgent, but they've directed it to the wrong goal. Not bad – a good attempt. It says, "It's now or never, come hold me tight. Kiss me, my darling, be mine tonight." Why tonight? We say, "kiss me, my darling, be mine for eternity!" Because you're telling God to kiss you with his lips of fire and transform you! The alchemy of total transformation. "Oh God, my darling, my beloved, tear me asunder, if you must, but save me from the evil gust. That's one of my poems Narsimha Mahadev to Sri Yuktsewar. So, you have to transform it to God.

It was a good idea, but it's a temporary, fleeting idea in your songs, and the culture is built through your songs, social activities, etc. I'm here to deepen your culture because you have been deceived by an evanescent culture. I give you something more permanent and something more true. And I'm not shy about going into your songs and giving you the real meaning. It's now or never, come hold me tight. Oh, God, hold me tight. I wilt not let thee go till thou tells thy name to me. And I will rest and fight with thee the whole night. That's Jacob. He wrestled with the angel, and he said, "I'll not let you go till you tell me thy name." That's how it should be, your fight, your wrestle and tussle and bustle and everything should be for God. All your energy should be directed to God. So, when you pray, you have to change the gestalt and turn it towards God. They're such beautiful songs. So from the love songs we sing to human beings, let's divert them and sing them to the permanent lover. One by one your relatives will be taken away from you. One by one your lovers will be taken away from you. Your aunt has died, your uncles died, your grandmothers died, nanny, this thing has died, so and so's sister. You're seeing it every day. The boyfriend breaks, the girlfriend breaks. Nothing is permanent. Everything is subject to disease, decay, and death. Everything that is created is evanescent and is changeable. Why not invest your love in something that is everlasting? Invest in everlasting love!

Part VII
Experiences

Yogiraj Gurunath Siddhanath

Preparing for the Experience of Truth

In today's satsang, I would not only like to tell you about the sacred and spiritual science of Kriya Yoga, but also prepare you and try to give you an experience of the uniting force of prana and an al encompassing experience of the unity of Human Consciousness.

Shift your consciousness from your mind to your heart. Do not listen to me thinkingly; listen to me feelingly.

You are not this house of flesh and bone. It is your birth right to understand that you are not this house of flesh and bone which sleeps, decays and dies. You are immortal consciousness, lord of the earth and the skies. Awake, oh sleeping image of God and realize that you are not this house of flesh and bone which sleeps, decays and dies. You are immortal consciousness, lord of the earth and the skies. It is toward this realization that many people have practised many kinds of yoga. The delusion that we are in has to be removed by the practise of these yogas. Practice feeling your body speck and your I-am-ness melting away with your vast infinite Awareness.

If you want to reach the highest truth, then you must get rid of all intellectual egoism – that I'm a knowledgeable man, that I am a great scholar, and I did this and I did that. So, the intellectualization of spirituality itself is an ego.

You can become the conqueror of life and death if you sincerely practise Kundalini Kriya Yoga and Raj Yoga of Infinite Awareness.

A Master Consciousness
An Alchemy of Total Transformation

When you blow the thoughts out of our minds, you do the silence, do you get a taste of them before you blow them away?

Thank God, thank God, I don't. Even when I do the Dreamweaver in the night – the chakra surgery Dreamweaver – I don't want to know what I've dealt with in each individual and all. All that have been transformed already, the bad and negative karma which has been neutralizes, let bygones be bygones and let's think about the positive light of God. It's even being done now, because if you are sensitive to me now, my main nature is not to think anything, but just to melt in a certain knowingness, you know, when I am awaring consciousness. So when I aware your consciousness, you will, many of you who are intent upon me, either looking at me or trying to listen to me, or feel my mind, will see that your thoughts have totally stopped. Even now I'm not doing anything, but your mind is very calm. There you are. It's a happening thing. An alchemy of Total Transformation.

You see, the Sun does not have to make a special blast of energy or sun rays to give us the warmth. It just comes up in the morning, and by the virtue of its being, and its radiance, we're feeling the warmth. So, a Master who's already there provides the virtue of his Consciousness. When that Consciousness gets into your thoughts, which are the basic source of all disease, delusion, and error, your mind also becomes transformed. And you feel that the trivial things of the world, they are not worth thinking of dissolve.

My consciousness, by my being here, exhausts your mind of all thoughts. The thoughts dissolve, because thoughts are the disease. It is from thoughts that all diseases and all sorrows arise. When I give a talk or give a lecture, I never think. ;.;The talk is always from awareness. My talk springs from no-mind. It springs from, the consciousness, not the mind. And it's your collective thoughts which make me speak what I do. So if you tune into me, if you tune your minds to my awareness, the moment you are tuned in, your thoughts will be dissolved. There will be no thoughts. Even though I am talking, you are not thinking. Consciousness is the mother of thought.

These are ineffable. We don't have any other words for them. But it's a state of blissful awareness, because you don't need to think. You don't need to agitate your mind. Thinking is agitation, movement. When you think, the molecular particles in your mind go to and fro. Molecule means that which goes to and fro. To, fro. To, fro. To and fro. To and fro. It's not necessary, because what you want, you have got. The tranquillity that you wanted, you have. So why think of anything else? You can just be like that.

Meditate Share Care

Even if I say Oh, la dee da, dee dee dum, you will have the transmission. So in actuality, you will be the people teaching. I will be the one talking nonsense and transforming. You can only teach. You cannot transform. I will talk nonsense – that's my prerogative Nonsense is the sixth sense, beyond the five senses. It makes no sense to the physical five senses, but it's beyond - beyond the normal, logical, digital brain. So it's nonsense. So, you don't have to grasp what I'm talking about. You have to grasp the transmission and how it's bringing a change. How this Divine madman is slowly making you into a Divine madman. It was just like this person in a prison. They said, "Come on now, you're perfectly cured. You're out of the lunatic asylum." He said, "No, no. Let me be here. Don't tell anyone that I'm okay. There's a bigger lunatic asylum outside these prisons walls. I don't want to go there!" So, in life we can't say whether those mad after money are crazy or those after God.

That's why the yogi is a recluse in his cave in the Himalayas. Why do we come to this little space? So that we can rest and relax, dissolve all our stress, and vent out all our fear and anxiety, but in the proper channelized way. It's good to vent out. You can do it any way. You can do it anyhow. But you have to move on. Time is fleeting. And you can only move on by practising Yoga sincerely and on the other side giving what you have learned. Sharing and caring with humanity, because they are a part of your larger Self. You cannot do without them. You cannot selfishly say, "Oh, I'll go ahead and give that fellow the slip." This is not business, you know, where you can do your Machiavellian tricks, and send your head-hunters and kidnap wise CEOs from one company and put them in another company. This is not that game. The more you give, the more you get. Honesty is the name of the game.

You know, all you people have a shield and you're very uptight, because you feel that if you're open-hearted to the world, the world shall eat you up. But that will not happen. If you are proper. If you have nothing to lose, everything to gain. Let go!

But how can I still my own mind and maintain equanimity?

This will take many, many years of Kriya practice as you breathe away at your genome and DNA, and your desires are slowly dissolved. Then, slowly, the thoughts will melt away.

Because Gurunath can do it effortlessly, anybody can do it? Who do you think Gurunath is? Is he some fellow on the road, kicking stones into the lake? Who is Gurunath? He has spent years to master the mind in his former lives, and you want it without making an effort? But I give you a present sometimes of my own mind – I give the cake of my own no-mind to show you what state of Awareness, or what state of no thought, I exist in. No pain, no fear, no tension. The thoughtless peace I experience is God.

But all of you can achieve this state. It's not difficult if you practice sincerely. The uninterrupted yogic effort to maintain equanimity of mind still awareness in Samadhi - it's not easy, because of your irregularity of practice.

Allow Yourself To Be Healed!

I can make you experience it as you go along the days more and more specifically. I'm just requesting you to be more receptive in the sense that you should be have the heart of a child – joyous, light and receptive. Not an inquiring or an intellectual mind. If you have a mind, then the heal or cure doesn't take place. So, when you have this receptive mind, then I can work with you. I may come and work with you tonight in your dreams, which I can easily do. I've got a lot of adjustments to make. Seeing the way, you all are sitting, surely, I have a lot of work to do tonight with your spine. Thank God that the beds are pretty stiff, that saved me a lot of work, but I have to work. My work is a ceaseless work – it's non-stop, night and day, 24/7.

And when I empower you, some of you feel it more. You feel a lightness of body, a freshness, and a joyousness of heart. You forget your tensions and leave your stresses behind. When you get all these feelings, I don't take the credit for all this, but let me tell you since I'm connected with you from past lives, I have to take this responsibility. Definitely a major portion of me is seeping through your heart and mind. But even though I'm doing that, it's up to you to allow me to do it. Are you allowing me to heal you? Are you allowing yourself to be healed? You must relax and allow yourself to be healed.

Now that your children are being looked after by people at home, there is time for you to relax, and take the greatest gift on Earth. You have the greatest gift on Earth, but you cannot tap your source. The fountain of youth lies within you, and yet you are hungry and starving and suffering and quarrelling – for what? Because you don't look within. Your mind is always engaged. You're always instructing and planning. You're planning this, you're planning that, and you're strategizing. So when are you going to live your life? Live it now. This is IT.

And therefore, live your life now and just be. "This is the moment; I'm going to receive every word of Gurunath. I have faith that at the next word he speaks, my pain will go away." I promise you, it will go away. "Gurunath, you spoke, and my pain went away only seventy-five percent." Dear sir, the twenty-five percent was the obstruction of your subconscious mind. I tell you – the mind which is undisciplined and which is in "I am-ness" – an egotistic mind – is the real Satan. That is Satan.

The Master is like the Pulsar Star: He's pulsating all the time. You can see, many of you – you're advanced people coming in for an advanced course, and definitely you've developed to a great degree clairaudience, clairvoyance, premonition, intuition. All of you have it to various degrees. And if you see the seven-coloured aura of the Master, you'll be able to see very clearly the rainbow-coloured man. The Master is always that. But firstly, you see the white cottony gold and that is the energy transmission of vibrations which seeps into every cell of your body and which goes into every wounded and hurt portion and heals it. But you must allow yourself to be healed. You're not allowing yourself to be healed because you are listening to me intellectually. Don't listen to me intellectually. Just relax, lean back, and feel me out. If you miss my words, it doesn't matter. Hear my words. Feel the flavour. See the flower. Not the intellect. Then the healing will take place.

The transmission is definitely happening spontaneously without any effort of mind. You will magnetically attract it to that portion of your body or your suffering emotion or your mental trauma or stress and I promise you, the sky is the limit for a receptive person. The sky is the limit! You can do it! The Good Lord does it; the Master does it.

So, the transmission is the velocity with which the pranic energy, or the kundalini energy called shaktipat, travels from the Master to the disciple. So, then, when this travels during their Kriya, during their process of meditation, it helps them and empowers them to practice the great lifestyle of Yoga!.

United Nations Experiential Address For Earth Peace Through Self Peace

Oct 25, 2007

I bow to the indwelling spirit residing in all of us. If earth peace is to herald the dawn of the new age, let us all realize the soul cry – the global ethic that, at the level of consciousness, humanity is one. And let us all realize that humanity is our uniting religion, breath our uniting prayer and consciousness our uniting God.

The core essence of the public good is the soul consciousness of love, humility and peace. The core essence of global ethics is the soul consciousness of love, humility and peace. And therefore, the core essence of the relation between the two must necessarily be the soul consciousness of love, humility and peace.

The public good may be divided or categorized into two sections - one is the objective section and the other, the subjective section. The objective section entails not only the giving of economic aid packages, building of medical institutes, the giving of medical aid and building of hospitals. What is necessary, as Dr. Sharma has rightly said, is that we need this transformative process in the globalized systems of the world today and unless these globalized systems, that's the core which we call the buddhi – the intuition, the intelligence of humanity at large – unless this intelligence is brought out, which she is doing a great work, because she has not had the time to say all this, with people actually, practically, pragmatically transforming them as best as she can by practical means, by teaching them, by books, through educational means, by practically going out and learning, which is a great work, and I think that we must all give her the fullest support we can give her. This is very very important and a very good opening for both of us to work in harmony together.

The subjective public good, however, is to do with the transformation of the minds of the people. It's a subjective inward process which links up with the outer work which Dr. Sharma is doing. For example, the elimination of emotional suffering, the mitigation of mental stress, and the harmonizing of conflicting ideologies between the peoples and nations of the earth.

Now this may best be brought about by three practical methods, which I am going to suggest to you here. The first practical method is by the practise of a yogic science called Kriya Yoga introduced to us by the great Mahavatara Babaji. I have personally practised the science of the breath – I think you had also mentioned the breath and the breathing – but I am not recalling in what context, but it was a very, very close link to what I am doing and through rhythm, it is very important, you see. I had an educational poem for children which I will tell you briefly, although time is short, and I don't know, every time Dr. Emery raises his finger like this (simulating finger movement), I think it's timeout. I think he will give me thirty seconds more.

As a leaking vessel – this is changing the basic, the system, the stagnant system can be changed –

As a leaking vessel never can fill the waters of life so pure and still,
So distracted mind fails to retain wisdom's nectar and its brain
To ease disease of random mind, a remedy suitable we must find
A rhythmic breathing tension free, with concentrating sovereign key

So this is, if we rather than studying books and teaching children, if by yogic methods of concentration and absorption, we can improve the very instrument of the mind, it can become a crystal bowl to gather the gnosis of a supernal mind. That is, like Dag Hammarskjold said, that "it needs a spiritual revolution to bring about the change in the world." I second this. And we honour his words today. He is not with us, but his spirit lives with us today. He is the first man who was trying to link, although may be it appeared a hopeless task, what, fifty years ago or forty years ago, whatever, but today it's coming because of the efforts of Dr. Sharma, Dr. Emery, Martha being so cooperative with us. Of course initially when we started, we were skating on thin ice, but then I think it consolidated and then it became very good and you find we are here to love and live as oneness, the experience of which I am going to give you today. The means is Kriya Yoga. The second means is we are teaching to children, everywhere in towns and villages, the radiating of earth peace through self peace by teaching them the earth peace meditations, which is very simple. We are going about this work in our own way – we have no funding, we need no funding, and I was speaking to Dr. Sharma and she told me, don't do that because if they have funding, there will be little of arm twisting, so get the funds from people who flow, get the funds from people who are related to you and who do it from the heart, and I think that was a very good advice and I think I am going to follow that.

And the third method is what I am going to give you today, dear souls, is a very different and a unique way. I am going to directly share with you my soul consciousness, which you will feel as a still mind state of abiding calm. I am going to share with you my soul consciousness. We have been able to talk by your grace. Your receptivity today will determine, it's how receptive you are, to that degree you will receive the still mind state of soul consciousness. I will transfer my soul consciousness of a still mind state which you will feel as an abiding calm. You will ask me what good this does. This does all the good in the world. It's the sacred space. It is the language incomprehensible to thoughts and to words, but is still the language which will transform the world, and which will build the bridge between the pragmatic and practical work which Dr. Sharma is doing and the inner spiritual work which I am doing. My heart is filled with joy and I am laughing because I am feeling my oneness with you already and I hope that you will cooperate with me and get straight from words which guide and inform to experience which transforms. We have read the menu, let's eat the food. Bon Appetite.

So now, I am going to go in for the experience. I would like all you people, if you can come to the front, because it's an eye-to-eye contact – they say the eyes are the windows of the soul. The eyes are the windows of the soul. You can stand at the back if you want to. I would get a little back. It's going to happen very fast and you will be surprised at its simplicity. Please be relaxed.

You can stand and do it, it's wonderful. The further back you are, you will see many more things, but that's not the subject of today. I will like you all to drop all armour and inhibitions for the unspoken language which Einstein, Albert Einstein, talks of – that we need another language to bring about a transformation in this world. This language is subtle. Be aware of it. Do not sit thinkingly, dear souls – sit feelingly. Drop all inhibition and armour and be totally relaxed and tune to me. Form the bridge between your heart and my heart. Get ready for the paradigm shift, from words which advise and inform to experience which transforms. And I am with you, when I clap my hand, you tune into me, upon your tuning receptivity will depend on your experience. But I will do it more than once. When I clap my hands and say, "peace", the moment I say that, your thoughts will disappear and you will feel a still mind state of abiding calm. That's it – a still mind state of abiding calm. Be relaxed, drop all your inhibitions. I am breathing through your breath now. I feel myself expanding in your mind. Relax, drop the shoulders, sit tall, drop the hands, be relaxed. You can explore my mind with your mind, mind my awareness while I aware your mind. I will still it with the awareness of abiding peace and you are with me in tune. Beloved captive audience, form the bridge, be in tune and when I clap, you will have the still mind state. Thoughts will disappear and you will find an abiding peace. Ready.

[Claps and says "Peace"]

The eyes must be kept open. Explore my eyes. They are the windows of the soul.

Shift the consciousness from head to heart.

If you connect with me, mind dissolves into consciousness. Aware yourself into my still mind state as I share with you consciousness of an abiding peace, so essential for the existence of humanity.

Okay, come back to your normal state. I wouldn't like to say that, but doctors describe all of us rushing around Manhattan as mild middle-class neurotics. It's not a very nice thing, but neurosis is cured by this as we go into the still (mind state). I am going to do this again, dear souls. Drop all your inhibitions and armour. If you can explore, tune into me, don't do your thing, do my thing, which is nothing.

And that peace will arrest the ageing process of body cells and bring to light your inner consciousness, because as long as there are ripples of thoughts in your mind's lake, you can not see the moon of your delight. You cannot see the indwelling Christ, because the ripples shatter the image of the moon. So also, a mind which is full of thoughts cannot give you the image of the indwelling Christ. So therefore, this is the basic thing to soothe the mind, calm the nerves, so therefore, I am going to aware myself into your thoughts.

As you mind my awareness, I will aware your mindless and in this exchange, if it is empathy, you can call it, or of its sympathy, you can call it, or an inner synchronicity, you can call it. Let's do it together.

This time I will go subtler and subtler – with the wave of a hand, then with the blinking of an eye, and then with nothing. You will be so much in tune. Each time it will be like layering an extra coat of honey on your calmness. You will feel it more and more with the second, the subtler. Be in tune with me, explore me, do my thing. I am sharing with you the universal consciousness of a still mind state of abiding calm.

[Waves the hand]

We are bathed in one-another's consciousness. We are awared into our soul essence of abiding calm.

You are sharing the initial stages of the samadhi of a yogi – what his mind is like in god contact. You are sharing the fringes of his core essence.

Come back to normal. Say after me everybody: "At the level of consciousness, humanity is one."

[everyone repeats]

"Experience of soul consciousness brings about earth peace through self-peace."

[everyone repeats]

So now the final time I am giving it to you, the third time, it will become deeper. I will hold it for long, because it will rest your whole system. The body is never not at work. Every thought creates an electrochemical action which brings ageing to the body cells. And this is one of the ways, in this moment of time – the American Medical Association says so, not me – that every thought brings an electrochemical action which brings ageing. So if you are not thinking, there will be no ageing in that moment of time.

So here is the third time. To go for the third, you must be able to contact me eye-to-eye, because if you explore what I am thinking of, which is nothing, your mind will be transformed into soul consciousness. The answer lies within, as I have read in one of Dr. Sharma's main sayings. And the answer will come from within only if you are still of thoughts.

You must keep looking at me, if your eyes are burning, I will take away the burning with the rose water. I am going to take away the burning of your eyes, with the wave of the hand.

[waves the hand]

The burning is gone. The mind must be free. Now, be with me.

Sharing our soul consciousness is the highest purpose and the will to good of humanity. This is what we must bring down into the practical world, and seep it with the spirit of righteous virtue.

Okay, please come back to your state.

Thank you so much for being one at the level of consciousness. And this is the simple message. The other language, the other thoughts which Einstein was speaking about, is the language and thoughts of the soul, which will be recognized through your own being – through your own action and a will to good for earth peace through self-peace. Namskar.

Be as a Child of Five to Heal

Open the petals of your heart and
let the light and love pour through!
Honey drop and dew, honey drops and dew
This nectar of Life permeates me and you!

See, all my poems are educational. I want you to teach this to your children as soon as they get up – they must know this. Let the child go to the school – that's okay even though they are teaching the superficial stuff and not teaching the very stuff that holds the knowledge. The child sees the fairies and the elves – you are taking away his extra sensory perception, the higher intuitions. Somebody says the child is just small – she says, "Aha! I saw the fairy and

I am riding the back of the dolphin," but they tell her, "shhh... shhh, go to school now, take your bags." So, the fairy, which was very subtle, which was actually there peeping out from behind the tree, has disappeared from the daughter's mind because education doesn't teach you the finesse of life. I am a successful person in life. I have had everything – I have had education, I've done the business, I have proved myself. Let me get back my lost memories as a child. Who wouldn't want that? What a care-free abandon we used to have, tumbling down from the slopes of the grass. Bring me back those days!

I talk about bringing back my childhood days, being as free as a child, nonchalant and not worried about a thing in the world. You grow up into tension, disease, decay, and death. What is it we've grown up into? The true education is the purity of heart, and it is the instrument whereby education is made possible. Books can be bought at any time if you have a perfect mind, you pick up a book, qualitatively feel it, put it to your heart, and inhale. What you get, you get. Leave to God the rest.

Evolution takes place when the mind is like a child. You cannot be inhibited. If your emotions are inhibited, there is a repression barrier in your limbic system which we try to constantly educate you into relaxing. The moment that inhibition barrier melts, healing takes place.

Experiencing Divine Love

What is the process one must take to realize divine love?

Take the path you're already taking. Make an effort to realize divine love. Practice selfless devotion - Bhakti - without an agenda or motive. You cannot know divine love unless you practice coupled the science of Kriya Yoga. You will only know affection. Human beings know the lower aspects of love, which is lust, affection, parental affection, brotherly affection. These are pale shadows of the true love which only comes after the state of samadhi. (Bhakti Samadhi/Bhava Samadhi)

But if there's another book, "Feel Intellectual," nobody will buy that book. But they do need to feel peace. Okay, let's say sexy is the most important thing, because most people are interested in that. But at least peace of mind is second most important. Let's go for that. That's what's got by Kriya Yoga. And once you get into that peace, then you feel a love towards all humanity. Love is a very high thing. All of you are hearing me with a great lot of admiration, but you must convert this into action during the coming days. The science of the self is selfing into the Self. You have to break down all barriers and get to the basic experience that Humanity is our uniting religion. Then only we can get together.

Dreamweaver

What you must realize is that the Dreamweaver is a short mini-dream, but your life is also an actual dream until your burst the bubble of the veil, the waking dream of maya and your clouded mind enters into the sunshine of enlightenment!

The normal state of a person is tension, illusion, delusion, and error, since he works in a world of duality. As long as there are ripples of thoughts in your mind's lake, you cannot see the moon of your delight. You cannot see your in-dwelling Christ or Krishna or Buddha, because the ripples of thoughts in the mind's lake will deflect the image into a thousand fragments. It's the patches of negativity in our emotional body – all our hurt. People hurt. The world is always cheating one upon the other. The name of the great illusion is cheat. Everybody's cheating on one another. That's the name of the game. Everybody's happy and then, in a moment, they are sad. If you practice Kriya Yoga sincerely, your mind will be always of equal bliss. Transcending the emotional pendulum of joy and sorrow your mind will purify itself to a state of equanimity.

Unless you break the bonds of relativity, and transcend that in the Dharma-megha samadhi, you will not know the ultimate reality.

All these lives and deaths are the ascent of consciousness into subtler and subtler realms of divinity until you get to your Divine Self.

You can't miss the Dreamweaver – it's your sloppiness or your mistakes in which you don't do what I say – but the Dreamweaver is already happening in a waking state or dream state or causal state. For all of you simultaneously, I will enter your dreams and I will do the work for you, and you will feel that you are being worked on. I will correct all your chakras. That is a madman thing, okay? Those in the causal will feel that they are being worked on; those in the astral will find me in their dreams guiding them. I may hit you in the dream in one of the chakras, or I may bless you. Please don't mind it, because if there is a blockage, I have to hit in order to allow your consciousness to flow into your Super Consciousness, your True Self.

Sleep now. Get up at two o'clock in the morning and meet here. I will say hello to you. You can ask me some questions, we can do a little chanting, and then you go back to sleep. I go back to sleep, and I will begin my work. From the time you sleep now to the time you wake up at two o'clock, you are with me. Dreamweaver is starting, and then you sleep again. Until you wake up in the morning, the Dreamweaver is still carrying on. Even now it's carrying on. I'm working on the light tapestry of your karmas lodged in your chakras and your subtle bodies.

When I appear to you in the dream, I appear, but it is suppressed at times at the back. It's buried. You don't remember it. But when others tell their experiences like you had, then that pops up and the memory recall comes after some time. Initially you don't remember, so later as is bubbles up from the surface of the mind, then you say, "oh I also had one, I remember now." It is suppressed by the later casual work that is done on you, so I am giving you time for it to surface. That is why I am waiting with you to share this. By sharing this, we invigorate and inspire each other to work more diligently in practising Kriya Yoga.

The dreams are for the person to get rid of their stress or their emotional suffering. Maybe I don't get rid of that but get rid of whatever is coming in the path of your Kriya breathing, the flame. If anything is obstructing the flaming star, that obstruction has to be removed. So, this is very succinct and specific work for which I expect nothing in return.

So now people want me to come in their dreams and do some repair work on the astral bodies and causal bodies. If you want me to, I am in two minds whether I should come or not, but with some people, they had some stress and certain problems and I worked with their astral bodies in their dreams. They either see me in the dream or feel me in the dream. They get rejuvenated and feel their bodies and chakras have been worked on. The pain is gone, the heart is lighter, you have a spring in your walk, and you can breathe a fresher air. So when I work with you in the night, it's responsible work for me.

If any mind is attuned to an undifferentiated consciousness, then that mind by the virtue of its velocity shall gravitate itself out of light-mind-existence and aware itself into that consciousness to the degree of its attunement with that consciousness.

Tonight, there will be an effort to work and to relax your motor-sensory nervous system, your astral body, and all the nadis. This will be the endeavour. During these two and half days, I will, with the resonant frequency of my voice, be working on your chakras, cleansing your chakras, working on your astral body, evolving the spiritual body, and dissolving the mental negativity. I will be doing all this, so the more relaxed you are, the more you will be feeling this happening. So tonight, there may be dreams; there may be incidences; there may be a good sleep. Whatever it is, because the work of the energy is started and you will feel these energies going into different dimensions or you may not feel it, please be relaxed and open. There is a service to all souls and evolutionary work to further Human Awareness.

Ceremony - The Sacrament of Sacraments

Tonight, dear souls, in honour of the Divine, in honour of earth peace through self-peace, and in honour of your souls, we perform this sacred fire ceremony which is as ancient as the hills. This is to align us all with the upcoming events beginning from 2012, 2013 according to the great Indian calendar, and ending 2700 when the Kalki Avatar the Second Advent shall come in a manifested form. This is to align you for that event so that there is peace and love in your hearts; we can spread it to humanity, and avert whatever crisis is to be upon us or not upon us. Irrespective, we praise the Lord.

Now shall be the invocation of the fire god, Agni Vaisvanara. The fire god stands for the eternal witness and is the messenger from man to the devas, to the demigods, and to the Divine One Himself. The original idea in the Indian pantheon and in the Indian spiritual practices is to invoke the flame. The Divine Spirit of the Elements fires the invocation fires of the Angelic Hierarchy. They will be present in the flame of the sacred fire.

To the south will be the earth element. The earth element represents Yama and the angel Azazel and is the first of the flames. The next flame, represents water and is known as Venus.. The third flame, will be the flame to the north and is the one represented by Mercury He represents fire and the sun. Then, in the eastern direction is Mars our fire. In the Indian Pantheon, it is the Lord This is the fourth flame. And in the centre is the fifth flame represented by Jupiter.

So, these are the five flames which are representing the five elements of nature. So, it's earth, water, fire, air. In the centre is Pater Ether, which is Space represented by Jupiter. So, these are the five flames. These are the native elements, which are represented in the Panchagni, the flame, which will bless you, give you their love, their wisdom, and their power. The fire element will take your message to the Divine Himself. And remember my words, what is the desire that, by desiring, all other desires are satisfied? God is that desire through which all other desires are fulfilled. We get to the source. It is the Divine Consciousness, and with this I begin the invocation of the fire.

Remember that a lot of negative karma is going to be burned. All negativities. Today is a sacred night – don't worry about the obstacles. Be patient and they shall be removed.

I'm invoking the fire god. Vaishvanara is the sacred fire god of the angel Rafael. The home fire of every family, when the home fire is lit you get food and warmth, and life is brought. So, for every householder, every person staying in society, the sacred fire is the eternal nourisher. He nurtures you, and from time immemorial lost, from the night of prehistory, the fire has ever been a friend of the man. If misused, it could be an enemy too. So, let us pray to the sacred god of fire, Rafael, the Agni, the Bhrigu and Kubera.

The Sacred Fire Ceremony

Now two by two you may come up and when I say "Swaha", offer your sacred desires into the flame. Offer your sacred desires into the flame. Two by two.

So, the first one is for God. Let me dissolve in Thee. Let me die in Thy Love. First is God, pure spirituality. What He represents within all of you. Second is any desire. When I say swaha each time you should put it in the blazing, pure, divine, and naked fire – blazing in your heart and blazing in the heart of humanity. May there be love and peace on Earth and goodwill to all mankind and humankind and womankind. Om Namah Shivay.

The blazing fire in the heart of humanity is in your hearts. May there be goodwill on Earth and peace and love for all humankind. So, first desire is God, I don't want nothing. I only want You, to dissolve in Your Love, pure spirituality. Second one is whatever you personally desire, but the first desire will fulfil all the rest.

1-First Swaha (Fire offering) To realize God alone.
The first is God, Thee for Thee alone O Lord, nothing else but Thee. Let me dissolve in Thee; I ask no more. O Lord, the whole world is but a dream in front of Thy Majesty and Glory.

2-Second Swaha (Fire Offering) Any Mundane Desire
All your negativity is being eliminated. May you find love and happiness and practice the right path. Breathe God through your breath. Ask in your oblation to dissolve your difficulties etc.

Now, the first desire will be Lord I want nothing from this world. When you want nothing, He gives you everything. When you want everything, He gives you nothing. We do not understand His ways. So, first is purely for God alone.

Don't dust your hands in the fire. It's the sacred Pentecostal flame. Keep the rice in your hands. If it sticks to your hands keep the rice in your hands.

Take the blessings. Put it on your head. Cup your hands and blow it to your loved ones if you want to. That's the open-flamed fire – you'll feel the effect immediately in your heart because the flame is Spirit. It's spiritualized. All the five Archangels are there – the big daddies who pull all the strings of our destiny. Connected through the five elements they come. It's a great science. They shrunk to a candle now in the church – it should be the open fire.

You'll feel the weightlifting. Be open and tune; you'll feel the lightness immediately. Walk on the clouds. Go to cloud nine.

If Thou art with me and the world is against me, I am the king of the universe, O Lord. For Thee and Thee alone, O Lord. So therefore, if I worship Thee from fear of hell, then burn me in hell, O Lord. If I worship Thee for the gain of paradise, exclude me thence. But if I worship Thee for Thine own Glory, withhold not from me Thine eternal Glory. Allakh Niranjan. Adesh.

Okay, now the last one is the purnahuti (Complete Oblation) into the Sacred Fire. Everybody stands up. Purnahuti. Now, you have to remember, what is the desire which desiring that all other desires are fulfilled? God is that desire. I'm not giving any of you Hamsas a material desire. God is that Source tapping through which all other sources are fulfilled.

All the Archangels, the Heavenly Elohim of the Pentecostal Flame, Michael, Gabriel, Rafael, Uriel, and Zadkiel, are all blessing us to take our desire for God, who knows best what we want and is fulfilling it. Now you can go back and sit. Take the blessings on top, put it on top of your head, and then cup your hands and blow it to your loved ones. You'll have to do it thrice.

This is the sacred ceremony of the fire. This is the original from where the idea of the Pentecostal flame came. The Pentecostal flame originated from the five elements – Indra, Varuna, Yama, Kubera, and the central Pater Ether, Brahma-Sarasvati.

So, this is the sacred fire because we believe the tongue with its spittle and its saliva cannot reach the God in ordinary prayer, but if it is chanted through the medium of fire, the fire is pure. They believed this in the ancient of days – seven thousand years ago – when Lord Ram performed the famous Yagya, the Raja Sur Yagya. Now all that is left are these little candles you see by the pool – that's all we have; it's shrunk to that. Where you see the fire flaming free in your heart, burning up your disease, burning up all your disease, burning up your evil karmas, and setting you free in the free flame of God, it is freedom from within. I pray to the Divine and all my love and blessings are with you. May we grow as a family. We are no religion except humanity, and as humanity we can grow and live in peaceful coexistence. Even if one of us, one of the arms of the Cosmic Man, is injured or damaged, it will hamper our efficiency towards Divine Realization.

Yogiraj Gurunath Siddhanath

Earth Peace Meditation

Therefore, let us pray for the peace of the earth by doing the Earth Peace Meditations. First, we make the humming sound, and we transform ourselves into the moon. Inhale love and watch me. I become the full moon. I radiate love for earth peace through self-peace. I inhale love. I do this thrice. Then I transform myself into the sun and explode. I transform myself into the sun. I fill myself, my heart, with six billion seven hundred million swans of love. I raise my hands, look up to the skies, and when I say explode, you explode these loves. Those who don't understand love by gentle ways must get love through the lightning path that will shatter their hatred. Love will shatter their hatred and we pray the Good Lord makes the world a better place to live in.

You must open the portals of your heart and therefore transform into love three times and then on the fourth time, you raise your hand and let the six billion seven hundred million missiles of swans explode in every human heart because that's the population of souls on this planet, so no one is left and do it with the full force. Keep doing it until you feel satisfied or until I put my hands down.

The explosion must be good – when you get into the sun explode the love of the sun. It's the spiritual seventh sun which we call Shiva. The spiritual sun shall explode for peace and love with all its power and all its splendour into the hearts of six billion seven hundred million souls of humanity.

How do you shrink it? You visualize Google Earth. Shrink the size – shrink the earth to the size of a baseball because you can't bombard the earth with love if it's too big. Your concentration will be scattered. So, to get your concentration together, shrink the Earth to the size of a baseball.

You're all experts, so I have to speak in your language now. It's the new age. You are already the sixth sub-race. From here, six hundred years hence when your soul incarnates, you will be the chosen ones who will be picked for the super-human race to enter Shambhala, the White Island. The King, the Arthur, the Vikramaditya, the Moses will come in all His splendour and take you with him for this new evolution. The Great Lawgiver, Vaivashwat Manu, Moses, Yukteswar will come. He will come. His forms are many. Yukteswar can take a million forms and appear before you even at this ceremony. Don't doubt his power; don't doubt his strength.

And now in the name of the Divine Ones, in the name of the Second Advent of Maitreya Krishna, Maitreya Christ, hold your hands and fill your hearts with love. Inhale love. You are the full moon – radiate love for earth peace. Radiate for earth peace through self-peace. Through your hearts and fingertips and your eyes and everywhere, your love is radiating. Still yourself, find your centre of gravity in your heart and your third eye. Fill yourself with explosive love. Transform yourself into the sun. Shrink the earth to the size of a baseball in front of you. Fill your heart with six billion seven hundred million swans for each soul on earth. Raise your hands to the sky, inhale love, explosive love, inhale. Remember the swans go like missiles to every heart of humanity. Spread your fingers out. Explode!

May there be goodwill on earth and peace and love to all humankind. O Divine Consciousness, give us Thy Love so that we may distribute it, spread it amongst all humankind. Give us Thy Wisdom so that we may disseminate it amongst all humanity. Give us Thy Truth and Power so that we can be empowered to bring about a change in this world where all can live in peaceful coexistence. Om.

New Sixth Root Civilization

My service to you is to lift you into the state of soul consciousness above meditation. I want to explain to you that this is a state above meditation. You are sharing my trance, my samadhi. Just the peripheral range – this is all I can give. I can pour forth my life to serve you as my larger self. And when this transformation happens, an evolution of quantum leaps take place. Every time your mind goes into a thought free state, the work is being done towards evolving a better humanity – a brave new world. This is an alchemy of total transformation and they have asked me how this evolution will take place en masse to millions and billions of people. It cannot take place at the physical level, but at the astral celestial level, when we enter the dreams of millions and billions of people and stop their mind – their gunas – the temperaments of their mind are transformed into a higher consciousness and that's how the evolution takes place. Instantaneously, within a fraction of a second, billions of people can be evolved slowly but surely without damaging their celestial astral system of chakras and the psychic nerves has to be persevered because that is their future. That's where they won't have mobiles, they won't have computers – it will all be within them. If they want to show a film, they'll show it through the third eye. If they want to communicate. They will receive all radar and normal messages in the Heart Chakra and generally in the chest areas etc! they'll tap this ear and they'll hear it from this ear, and speak from the other ear mentally. Spiritual messages will go through the third eye. This is the evolution of a future humanity, the raw material of which are you. And to refine you and and evolve you as the work of God, we are sent here.

You are the selected echelon. This is not the common people – this is selected people. You are spiritually more advanced, whatever you say. But you tap the widest of source from humanity and then connect it with Divinity. So that's the whole idea. Whatever the peripheral desires or results may be, those are human desires and results which are natural for human motivation to go on, but the Divine is involved in there. So whoever is making such an effort, I am sure all of you are making an effort. There are other people who are making many such efforts. So give all yourselves a hand for helping in the peace and evolution of humanity. Through Earth Peace Meditation, Surya and Kriya!

Part VIII
Miscellaneous Topics

The Practice of Kriya Yoga – What You Need to Know

How long do we have to practice Kriya Yoga? How much Kriya Yoga do we need to do for it to be effective and for us to see results?

There were two ladies. In India we have a common tap in the villages, and they took all their dishes and they started washing their dishes by the tap. One lady said, "your utensils are shining, and you've finished and I'm still scrubbing away. What is the problem?" So, the other lady said, "your utensil has a lot more grease on it, and masala, so that will take a little bit more time to come out." So, in Kriya Yoga, who gets more enlightenment or progress depends upon how much masala of karma you have to wash out. Some people have less karma – less action and reaction. Less negativity. So, they can see the inner light of God quicker than those who have more karma. They are both evolving at the same speed, but since the grime – the grease of their karma – is not being cleared as quick as the other person, he sees it six months later and the other person person sees it six months earlier.

So the speed of Kriya Yoga will depend upon two factors – how much negative karma you have – the more you have, the longer it takes – and secondly, the degree of concentration applied to the spinal breathing – the sadhana. It is very specific and gives you mathematical results. Half a minute of spinal breathing, concentrated spinal breathing, is equal to one year of natural spiritual unfoldment. So the evolution depends on the degree of concentration and how much karma you have. The more karma you have, the longer it will take. And vis-a-vis concentration, the deeper you concentrate, the faster will be your evolution. Suppose the man who has more negative karma concentrates more than the man who has less karma. They might get enlightened at the same time because his evolution will be twice as fast due to the degree of concentration applied.

How does Kriya Yoga help in our daily life, which is busy, full of tension, stress, satisfaction, and unrest? How will it help me to lead a better life and bring a balance between work life, family, and myself?

Kriya Yoga will do just what the question asked – that is the purpose of Kriya Yoga. Thank you.

There are so many forms of yoga. Why Kriya Yoga called the lightning path?

So this is a bit of an in-depth question. Since there are many yogas, why Kriya Yoga and why is Kriya Yoga called the lightning path? The great master Gyanavatar Sri Yukteswar here developed a science called cosmic astrology and he had placed the twelve signs of the zodiac within the spinal cord and the shada chakras – six-by-six polarity all in the spine. When you concentrate and you make a microscopic picture of the macrocosm of our solar system within your spine, the speed of your evolution evolves because you are travelling at a tremendous speed. When you focus your concentration, you travel faster and faster, so that you can travel at the speed of light.

This is the secret of yoga. And those master who bring concentration to vanishing point – travel at the speed of light – their mass is infinite. The great masters like the Lord, Sri Krishna, Prabhu Ram Chandra, the Gyanavatar Yukteswar, Yogavatar Lahiri Mahasaya, Bhagwan Patanjali, Bhagwan Vaivaswata Manu have all fulfilled this awful condition. And great people like Isaiah, Ezekiel, Moses, Jesus, and Elijah – they are all very advanced yogis and have fulfilled this. They all reincarnated – even Zarathustra in this former life and latter life. The great twelfth Zarathustra incarnated as VedaVyas and then Gautama Buddha with Pythagoras as his disciple.

So, these are great souls. The degree of their concentration increases the speed of their evolution. And when your evolution goes towards the speed of light, obviously in half a minute you can do one year of natural spiritual unfoldment: the man who goes for his daily church service and prays and does Hare Krishna or Hare Rama or does many techniques – Art of Living. All good techniques, but when he does scientific Kriya – when he focuses his mind – that person will take one year what the Kriya Raja Yogi will do in half a minute.

So, this is for eagle hearts who cannot wait. This is for people who cannot wait. They don't want wealth and name and fame. They want the Divine.

> God, I'm burning in my love for thee.
> Eternal infinite,
> I cannot rest in peace now
> Till I do become thy light.

If a person is so intense, then he will surely see the Lord, and this is the right way. This is for eagle hearts and not for tortoises who go slowly by. So, it's an individual evolutionary thing. Like I made a poem in Farsi:

> I do not want to become a beggar nor an angel
> I do not want fame, nor money
> the diamond scepter of the kings
> Just give me thy awareness, oh Lord
> Because having Thee,
> I will have the universe.

Does Kriya Yoga bring healing, peace, joy, fulfilment in life or does it bring transformation where practitioners will ultimately leave their current lives and become a hermit living in the jungle or mountains?

Jungle or mountains . . . I'm going to take away everything you like – from your glass of bear to your nice family life to all your Richy Rich money to your name and fame – everything I'll take so that nobody will come for yoga. Listen, the Kriya Yoga I've come to teach is called the Householder's Kriya Yoga. It's not the very supernal Kriya Yoga, which is a blazing light, but it is the Kriya Yoga meant for the householder. And when you leave your cigarettes and leave your drinks and wine, you will have no trouble because it will automatically fall away by your own inner decision. You will not feel like smoking or earning money by deceit or greed as your system gets cleansed and purified by your yoga practice. So it's an inner happening which takes place. The flower falls when the fruit appears. The flower of your desires will fall and the fruit – the results of Kriya Yoga – will appear. And you will know that God is the ultimate joy, the ultimate wife, the ultimate husband, the ultimate father, the ultimate mother, the ultimate child, and the ultimate of everything. Because God is the goal of everything you aspire for. Seek God first; everything else will follow.

So, you don't have to leave and go to the jungle. You don't have to go to the Himalayas. In your house, in a simple way, you can practice this technique and still progress spiritually fast, having the love of your grandchildren, your wife, your husband, your father, and your mother. And gradually you will move into this and they will also get a happy life due to your vibrations. I am a householder Yogi and am leading a very contented life.

This is a great fear in the mind. Don't have fear. It is simple and easy. Anyone can do Kriya Yoga and you can do it as a householder yogi. This is the new gift from Maha-avatar Shiva-Goraksha-Babaji, from the Himalayas. Please avail of this and actualize the essence of your life. It is very necessary for us to do this.

Guruji, who can practice Kriya Yoga? Can children practice Kriya Yoga?

All those who are breathing. All those who breathe as human beings. All the human beings who breathe can practice Kriya Yoga.

Now, can children practice Kriya Yoga? Yes, children can practice Kriya Yoga from the age of twelve. Twelve is a suitable age at which I personally think their mind can get steady and they can get on the path. After he has crossed the age of twelve, it will help him to do what he is already doing better. By concentrating on his breath, he will also be able to concentrate on his examination papers and on his studies. So yes, of course, you can teach them at the age of twelve. You're welcome – it's very simple.

What Is Yoga?

Yoga is an inner ascent through ever more refined and ever more expanded spheres of consciousness to get to the god essence which lies at the core of your own being. Once you contact this divine in-dweller, you can contact the universal in-dweller.

We have a good support system. Wherever we go in United States of America, or Switzerland, or Italy, we have teachers who can give you the support and teach you and guide all newcomers. In India also, we have good support system. Of course, principally I am not a teacher, since I do not teach. A Master does not teach – he gives the direct experience. You see, the teacher teaches very systematically in an organized way. The Master catches you and shakes you and wakes you up. I am a waker, mover and shaker!

You give the transmission and breathing through our breath. Doesn't that take tremendous amount of energy from you?

When I do this, the effort taken to breathe through one person and the effort taken to breathe through ten million people is the same for me. There is an expenditure of energy, but it multiplies itself because it is just my larger self and, if the circuit is complete, the energy flows as in one person, just like we are all breathing. I am not tired because you are breathing. So also, I am just connecting the breath. Now you are breathing individually like this, up and down, and I am connecting it in a horizontal circle to prove the point that the whole of humanity is tied by the self-same chord of love through breath. That's the purpose of this exercise – unity of humanity is the purpose of this exercise.

What is the reason for doing the Hamsa breath and the three lotuses we are using – the navel, the heart, and the third eye?

Chakras, because it activates certain bases of energy which we have already been working on and which humanity is already evolved from. Technically, I meant to work on the sex centre, the heart centre, and the third eye centre, but we work on the navel centre – pulling it up to the navel centre, the heart centre and the third eye centre. They are the three Granthies. The knots are actually at the base of the spine, which is the Brahma Granthi, which is partially opened in everyone. That is the first knot which comes as an obstacle to the further growth of spiritual energy. That knot has already been loosened by the evolution of humanity at large, but not fully. We still have to work on it. For that, I give individual practice by perineum pressure.

The navel centre makes your mind very steady and constant. So, I do that instead of working on the sex centre, since if I give transmissions on the sex centre, everybody will be sexually activated, and this will create a lot of misunderstanding all over the world. We don't want that to happen, because people are not matured enough to understand this advanced technique of evolution. So when you work on the navel centre, it pulls up the sexual energy to the navel centre and that centre helps you to steady your mind. The parameter of the steadiness of mind is the basis for all successful yoga. So, the navel centre is very important, and it's just as good for digestion - Saman Pran. Good to balance the mind.

Second is the heart centre. The first alchemy transforms passions to emotions – the sex centre is lust and navel centre is passion, so lust and passion are grouped together in the navel centre and transformed. Lust transforms into passion, then the passio-emotional nature comes to the heart centre, where the passio-emotional nature transforms to love. When it comes to third eye, love transforms into divine consciousness. This is the alchemy of total transformation.

In the real alchemy of total transformations, you are meant to breathe through all the seven centres, and I told you what all the centres are. The main centre at the bottom is lust for life, the urge to be and to exist. Your existence is in the root chakra, in the brain – the seven brains of humanity as we spoke about. That's in the root centre – your lust for life, the urge to exist, the urge to live on. The second centre is the sex centre – the centre of procreation of the human species, so that we may not die out. We procreate and make more of ourselves. It's a race against nature – the survival of the fittest in this harsh world. We don't want the human race to be wiped out, so there it is. The third, after this lust and this existence, you have the passion centre. This is the emotional centre. The highest emotion centre in the heart is love. Then love goes to the consciousness centre of third eye (agya). Love is transformed to consciousness and later it is transformed to divine consciousness in the transpersonal centre of the thousand petalled lotus. This is the reason why we do it in the three centres, because there are knots there. There are ganglia, and they have to be loosened for the evolutionary energy to flow up.

First the top of the head, then navel, then heart. Is there a reason for that?

This centre (top of the head) is just an invocation, called the great invocation. The great invocation is when we invoke the divine spirit of the rainbow-coloured light to flood our body. This is the temple of humanity. Great invocation -Avahayami! Avahayami! Avahayami! – so the great spirit comes and floods our body with rainbow coloured light. Then you choose the colours green, gold, and all the colours – the pearlescent colour here (at the third eye). So the green lotus transforms the passional nature – lust and passion to emotions. Then it transforms in the golden heart centre to love and love to divine consciousness. At the third eye, this is to invoke the spiritual energy. Before we start, we flood the whole body. We need the working material. The body is the car, but we need the fuel. Can you drive the car without petrol or without gas? So Shakti Energy is the fuel – the hundred octane elixir to transform your body car – and with that energy, we work. Green lotus, golden lotus, and pearl and swan. Is that clear?

What of Christ Krishna Consciousness, Christos-Narayan Consciousness and God-Shiva Consciousness

The Christ Consciousness is in our heart chakra and the Christos Super Consciousness in the Third Eye Chakra – and Shiva the Cosmic Consciousness. And beyond is located in our Crown Chakra. Christ is here (the heart centre) as the fully-blossomed Jivatma – the swan. The Christos is here (third eye), the Supreme Shiva-Goraksha-Babaji, Supreme Throne, the Throne of Sahasrara, So this is Paramatma – Christ consciousness –Heart Christos the third eye – Crown Chakra divine consciousness. I should say, the perfected human Divine consciousness of Christ. The Super Divine Consciousness, and beyond that, 'He about whom not may be said.' The difference between these consciousnesses is not of kind – it is of degree, if I may be permitted to use such imperfect words for such a perfect description. We are at a loss as to what we should use to describe these high states. But I think it's a fairly good idea I've given you.

How is it that the body is designed, so that Kriya is such an effective technique for evolution? It seems like it's too easy. Then, why don't they just make us enlightened right away?

You are! But the splendour of your soul is covered by the mud of your mind; wash it away by Kriya Yoga! It's all about sustained Sadhana and your inner soul flame yearning to be with your parent

The Reality of Kriya Yoga

Source, the Lord!

The advanced techniques are so not easy. It's a very gradual process. It takes life after life after life. Since we are a part of higher beings, they will not evolve us, but we will have to make our own efforts. Even though I am helping you as a Guru and a Master, you will have to get the hard-won gold yourself. You wouldn't like somebody else to run the Olympics, make him win the race, and you take gold medal. That's a shame! So, you need that self-pride and self-esteem to win the hard won gold by the sweat of your own brow.. It's not an easy method, but it is a simple process. You can progress. Everyone can do it. It is simple, and in a sense, it is easy, but it takes a long time. It can't be done in the wink of an eye. It takes lifetimes. This is a faster process, but still, it takes a lot of practice. It's not so easy for the restless ego-oriented mind, but it is a simple technique for the mature and steadfast mind to get to its own perfection.

They watch and wait. They cannot interfere in your evolution. You may not want evolution.

There is a story of a man who did a mantra and lot of meditation, and he did it powerfully. Actually, he went to his Guru and he wanted a mantra to contact the dancers of heaven Apsaras You know, in India, we have the beautiful fairies of heaven. They are known as Ramba, Urvashi, Menaka, and all this. He was enthusiastic and did a lot of sadhana to contact them. He overshot the mark and met Krishna and he said, "oops, I am sorry God, I didn't want to overshoot the mark – I wanted to go the paradise of beautiful women, where I could enjoy heaven." He overshot the mark in his enthusiasm to see the heavenly dancers. He didn't want moksha.

So, they don't interfere – they say you get what you want. There is the example – this fellow didn't want it. So, you have to practice on your own and not depend on others. You have to do it on your own. You see a mother seal teaching its baby seal to swim or a mother duck just pushes them with the wing, and they have to swim themselves. A child is born, they help it to stand, it tries to stand, and it falls again, but it has to make the effort to stand with its own willpower. So also, when you have to stand in the light of God, you have to do it by your own courage and willpower and strength. That is your self-esteem and that is your joy. What's the use of I keep breathing for you twenty-four hours a day? That's what you are saying – why don't you do it? I was doing it. I was breathing for you.

But if I do constantly, you will say, where is my glory? You stole my thunder, you'll say. And when God asks you, "is your enlightenment self-achieved?" then you will hang your head in shame. You will say, "no, my examination paper was written by someone else, and I got the certificate. We don't want that to happen, so you must make your own effort.

That's the way it is, but they are progressing all the same. Enlightenment is a great thing. Nobody has gotten enlightened – except, in America, everybody says everybody is enlightened. In India, we say nobody is enlightened. One Christ, just once in a while. Once in centuries there's a man called Gautama Buddha. He first incarnated as Vyasa, then Zarathustra, and then when he came as Siddharth, he was enlightened. We know of no other case after that.

When Karma Challenges, Do Kriya Yoga Practice

What can be done when the body is going through some physical karma that blocks any way of living one's life while also doing Kriya practice?

Well, that means you're working out your karma. Your obstacles have not come to you for no reason at all. God or his laws are not just random or unjust. His laws obey a perfect balance, a perfect system, where you're fitted into the jigsaw of your puzzle as you yourself have planned. So, what you're getting in your past karma is you're getting the good benefits of what you did in your past or you're getting the negative benefits of what you did in the past. So you yourself are to blame for your own joy and happiness and you yourself are to blame for your own difficulty and sorrow.

Now, where does Kriya Yoga come in? Kriya Yoga is the means whereby – it is the sovereign key – whereby you may open the doors of happiness to your future where you may overcome your negativity, overcome your difficulty. And even if you don't, keep persevering. Keep trying. Pranayama and meditation neutralizes your karma.

When there's pain that comes up in the physical body and there's obviously something that's not right, how can I make use of Kriya practice to help mitigate the pain?

Say "God, I'm trying to do the Kriya Yoga of Babaji, of God, that was given to me. But you have come as an obstruction to me. Oh Babaji, you have come as the pain. I bow to you and honor you, but please try to understand that it is your work that I am doing. Remove yourself as the pain from me so that I may practice the Kriya Yoga." Even though he is not coming as the pain – it is your own karma – just put the blame on him. Put everything on him, and then he will take the load. And many a time, it has happened that he has removed the pain. I tell you that it can happen, and it will happen. He has removed the pain. He has come to your help, and he will come always. And not only when he removes the pain of an individual – he will save the whole of humanity especially those of the path of Yoga

These are the Being who can bend the world matrix. They are the people who are the creators, preservers, and the liberators of many a humanity past, present, and future. It is in their power and glory in which we live and keep on living.

So, have faith. Things will pass. He will come. You, on your part, are an immortal soul. It's your body that is getting the pain. Tell him, either remove this pain or give me the power to detach and fly away from my body like a free bird – like the Hamsa swan – and taste of the eternal spirit of immortality. I will endeavor, I will strive to be in Thine Awareness.

I know it is easier said than done, but always have a try and you will get success. Nothing is a hopeless case. Nothing is done. There is no such thing as everlasting damnation. There's always hope. There's always the love, the power, and the glory of the divine ones to help you along the path. So take courage and keep practising.

Kriya Yoga and the Spine

It's very clear that the spine is a critical aspect of evolution, especially in yoga and Kriya Yoga, so what about people who

have injuries to the spine or sometimes people have an altogether deformed spine? How can they avail of the benefits of Kriya Yoga?

Definitely the spine is one of the main factors for the evolution of human consciousness, and the spine is used for the evolution of human consciousness because that is the direct path to express cosmic consciousness. If a man in his normal routine were to express cosmic consciousness, scientists and great yogis have found out that it would take a human being a million million years to express Cosmic Consciousness. But, if you use the lightning path, the Kriya path – the technique of the spine, it will make you go much faster, and you can do one year of natural spiritual unfoldment in half a minute of Kriya breath. That's the efficacy and efficiency of the simple but effective technique of Kriya Yoga.

Now, the second question is if a person has an injured spine. He will not be able to evolve as fast as a person who has a spine which is in good condition, but the spine has its subtle counterparts. There's the physical spine in the sushumna nadi, then there's the vajra nadi – the astral spine, then there's the chitrini – subtler than that and causal, and then there's the Brahma nadi, which disappears into no nadi – to pure consciousness. So those are availed of at times – the physical crookedness or injury or deformity of the spine can be overcome by a degree of concentration, going into the astral and causal spheres and doing your Kriya mentally there and still evolving. This is what can happen. So, do not be discouraged – onwards and upwards.

Kriya Yoga and Karma

You mentioned earlier that the downward flow of apana actually burns away negativity, so can you just explain a little bit more about the co-relation between Kriya Yoga and karma?

Kriya Yoga is the process of using your life-force energy to detoxify your system, rejuvenate your body cells, burn your past evil karma – those karma which are an obstacle in your upward growth, and evolve your consciousness. Now, in my work with people, what I do is this: when I transfer my consciousness in their prana and breath, I work in their spine and I work in the chakras. The destiny of man is in his spine; the karma of man is in his spine. So when the master takes his disciples and works on every center, meridian point, or chakra lotus, therein are lodged the chromosomes, the genes, and the DNA. Now, how Kriya works is that the gentle abrasion of Kriya works on the DNA. The DNA is like a nitrogen nub. These nubs have a film which can be unfilmed – the film of the motion picture of this life is on the DNA of your prarabdha karma in your spine. So when the gentle abrasion of Kriya comes, it unfilms the DNA – the nitrogen nub – and that portion which is not required or which hinders the spiritual growth – the forward march of the evolution of the soul – that portion or that obstruction is removed by the master in his Dreamweaver when he works with the Kriya breath of the disciple. The disciple himself in a general way also, by the gentle abrasion, works on the DNA and the genes of that prarabdha karma which is given to him in this life, and that karma is rubbed out by the gentle abrasion of the breath. The rough edges of the personality are rounded off until the gentle abrasion of the Kriya breath transforms every jiva into Shiva gradually using techniques of higher Samadhis as well.

But this is long years of practice – long lifetimes of practice. It's not a magic show – it's good, hard, diligent work. When you bind your mind to the breath, breath to the prana, prana to the soul, and the jiva to Shiva, then the effect is very, very powerful.

Kriya Yoga transforms every kankar into Shankara as it passes through the Samadhis.

There's a river called Narbada which everybody in India knows – the Narmada river – where every kankar is transformed into Shankara. Every kankar into Shankara. Because the gentle abrasion of the Narmada river smooths out the rough edges of every stone, making every kankar look like a Shivalinga and a Shankara. So also, the gentle breath of Kriya Yoga rounds off the rough edges of your personality and makes of every jiva, a Shiva of pure consciousness.

I love that, it's really nice. And I really love your poetry – the fact that you just flow with this, whether you're speaking in Hindi, in Sanskrit, or in English. How is that? Is it because you're really tuned into . . .?

Must be spontaneous.

Interview Q&A

Pranayama and Pranapat of SatGuru

So, it is always said that the quicker you breathe, the shorter your lifespan. The giant tortoise breathes four breaths per minute and lives for four hundred years; the elephant has sixteen breaths per minute, he lives for a hundred years. Man has about twelve and twenty breaths per minute; he lives for about eighty years.

I do not tell anybody to follow any religion. I do not anybody to be of a particular faith or creed. I tell them, just scientifically practise the Kriya Yoga with focused attention, and you shall reach the goal.

So, with Kriya Yoga, breathing in, of course, pure air which you will find in the early hours of the morning, you will oxygenate your system. It is a very healthy process of blood and lung purification.

We must share our spiritual wealth in experience and inform with everyone who comes. Talk is talk so practice as well!

So, when I transmit, my chaitanya prana in your pranic shwaz, to be technical, you've already been given anugraha. Anu means 'self' and graha means 'home' – you've entered your self-home by breathing with my breath. This is spiritual intimacy – when the master throws his breath and is breathing through the disciple, that is what is called closeness. Not just going and saying "hi" and hugging someone and all – still you're separate – but here, the breath and the prana and the chaitanya breath has been mixed, showing to humanity that we are one. Prana evolves humanity.

How does Kriya Yoga help our loved ones?

Okay, I want to ask you a counter-question: how will not doing Kriya Yoga help your loved ones? It would not help either way. The Yoga most importantly requires commitment from your loved ones and from you! Not doing it will not help you nor your loved ones but doing it would help you and encourage your loved ones to do the same. But the answer is even better – yes, it will help your loved ones if they are attuned to you, and you let them know, 'I am doing Kriya Yoga for you.' Definitely it is going to have a pacifying effect and it will give them a lot of courage and support. It's a good support system, and try to bring them later to do it, because it's a science and not a religion. It's a scientific technique that soothes the nerves, calms the mind, and detoxifies the whole system. It's the fastest method of detoxification. This Yoga is a lifestyle and not a religion. If loved ones can commit to practicing the Yoga then the benefits are maximum.

Mercury Shivlinga and the Surya Kavach

The Surya Kavach is the first Rejuven-Detox technique fills you with light and protection. It is to protect your body and to keep you away from accidents, premature death, and all ill-happenings, because the Surya is the king of the mandala – the rashi mandala is ruled by the Surya. It's common sense, because if there's no sunshine for two or three years, all life on Earth will die away. We are floating in the soup of the sunlight, and in him, we live and move and have our being. So Surya Narayana is our immediate God. The other Lord God you cannot see, but Surya you can see every day. He is our immediate God and sole life giver the ParamAtma of our whole Solar System.

You know what I would love to do? I would love to invite you to my ashram in the forest of the Sinhagad hills near Pune. It is a beautiful forest – we have deer and peacocks in season and it takes you five thousand years back in time because we have thatched huts and mud houses. And we have this temple. And you can stay there overnight – it's really wonderful. That's where I teach the Kriya Yoga and Surya Yoga, and it's very, very good – it's very rewarding. At Pune Ashram, you get to see the world's biggest akand Shivaling, made of pure Mercury (parasmani). That is in the temple, so you'll get the opportunity to meditate there and still your mind. It is a high samskara alchemical mercury Shivaling – consolidated mercury. And they say in the shastras that the paras-mani Shivaling, paradeshwar, is the highest Shivalinga which anyone can ever have – more than emerald; more than diamond; more than gold; more than silver. So we have one of the biggest parasmani Shivalings or the biggest in the world, which is akand and has eighteen samskars.

Yogiraj Gurunath Siddhanath

Tell us about the essence of Kriya Yoga

Kriya Yoga is a spinal process. It is breathing. It is called the sacred fire right of the yogi. There are two currents involved in the practice of Kriya Yoga. One is the pranic current which flows from the muladhara chakra to the agya chakra. It is upward and ascending. The other is the apanic current. It flows from the third eye down to the muladhara base centre. So, these two – the prana and apana currents – are utilized in the evolution of your consciousness.

But to prepare for this, you must do Hamsa vai-upasana before, which we call the baby kriya – vipasana, which they have mispronounced. Vai-upasana – just being a witness to your thoughts and breaths and do not think – this is the first stage, because this is a purificatory stage. Vai-upasana or vipasana, as they call it, purifies your mind, but Kriya Yoga evolves it from man the brute to man the man to man the god, all the while concentrating in the spine.

So, in this process, he does the fire ceremony of prana and apana, offering the inhaled to the exhaled breath and the exhaled into the inhaled breath. This is called "Pran-Apan Yagna" – Fire ceremony.

Now, let me explain to you what Kriya Yoga does, okay? He who offers the inhaled to the exhaled breath and the exhaled into the inhaled breath – he awakens his kundalini. That is why it is known as Kundalini Kriya Yoga. It is he who does the yogic fire ceremony, because kundalini herself is fire. And if kundalini awakens, what does she do? She destroys your ego. The yogi is enlightened. So, through the seven layers of kundalini, or even the third, fourth, fifth layer, he gets his partial states of enlightenment.

This is what Kriya Yoga does, and you, as you continuously breath long in your spine, are helping your shallow breath to extend itself with the result that more oxygen is collected in your lungs. Remember the lungs are the distillery of your body and your heart is the pump! If more oxygen is collected in your lungs, then the heart beats slower – that means less wear and tear for the heart. The heart beats fast to get more oxygen. So, when by Yoga you breath slowly there is extra oxygen and the heart beats slowly. The heart is the body pump – and when there is a preservation of the body pump, your cells are then kept in a spiritually magnetized condition, you live longer. The heart is pumping eighteen to twenty tons of blood a day – by Kriya Yoga you can reduce it to eight tons, six tons, three tons, two tons, to a few pounds, and still your body machine and be at total rest.

So Kriya Yoga – the spinal breathing – not only gives you enlightenment, but at the lower level, it gives you recuperative rest. All these techniques being taught are basic techniques compared to Raj Yoga – it is so deep. It recuperates and repairs your body cells. So what happens? If your cells are rested, anti-ageing occurs. Sorry ladies – I don't want to take your, if any of you have opened a beauty spa or something, I don't mean to take away your business – but this is Kriya without which Raj Yoga does not happen.

If you see a yogi, he will usually be glowing, and if you have a little clairvoyance or spiritual vision, you will see a light emitting from his face, his eyes, his body. Any yogi who can call himself a yogi must have these qualifications. So next time you see a sadhu– look for these things. You should see all these things and you should feel that. He should be able to throw his prana. That is the satguru who initiates you without moving from his place. That is a direction for you because in today's supermarket of Yoga and Yogis – many people are misled and disappointed. But there are the hallmarks of a true Yogi – that's how you know the yogi.

I enjoy positive emotions, but when the negative emotions come, that definitely disturbs me and disturbs my work. So, of course, I observe many meditations and all. With this yoga that you're teaching, can I burn quickly all negative emotions in me?

There are two factors in this. My first answer to you is, yes you can. Firstly, it will depend on the regularity of your practice – on your effort. Your regular effort, you see? The second is your karma. Some people have bad karma; some people have good karma. It's just Newton's third law of motion – every action has an equal and opposite reaction. So it depends on how many mini-traumas and mini-reactions you have created which are negative from your past and this life, which have coalesced into your collective subconscious. Kriya Yoga is a method of churning out this negativity and spewing out all the negative unconscious thoughts – all the toxins of the body. So, for this, you definitely have to do sat-tat abhyas. Now what happens in some cases is that, when a person starts, he gets so much negativity coming up, bubbling up, he says, "I was better off when I didn't do Kriya! It's going so bad; I'm feeling so depressed."

That's the test where you should not stop. Of course, if you need a little, you can stop for a few days and carry on – if you overcome that, then you are a victor. Then you will defeat all your negative emotions. A human being is a human being. You see, like we say, there's ups and downs in everyone's life – take it like a man. I think Kriya Yoga tends towards positivity and, yes, it's a question of time. The Master will give you the strength.

People came to me and they said, "can I get rid of negativity?" One fellow came and he got rid of negativity within the first twenty days. The next fellow took three months. The third chap got it done after two-and-a-half years. So they said, "why this difference?" I said, Kriya Yoga is like cleaning off the lamp glass – we have a lantern that gets soot in it, so if the soot gets thick, it takes more time to show the flame of positive life, and if the soot is less, Kriya Yoga cleans it quicker. So Kriya Yoga is the process of cleaning the lamp glass of your body and mind. And so, do not be discouraged – it must work; it has to work.

You know, I used to read about a Siddha – he projected his prana and other people are breathing through his breath. We read some things about Abhinav Gupta where he said one of the highest initiations is to breathe through the breathing of the disciple, which I give you. So, I said, is this to be given to the common public? But who knows whether they're the common public – they might be advanced souls of a past life. They've already done it.

Do you give initiations on mantra diksha individually?

Yes, if I feel it's necessary. The initiation consists of a very powerful mantra. The mantra comes from the heart and its ripples steady the mind. So Kriya Yoga itself is a great mahamantra.

I want to meditate starting tomorrow – what do I do?

Nobody can meditate – meditation happens as a result of sadhana concentration. What is sadhana? Kriya Yoga is sadhana. Sadhana is the practice of spiritual growth. You practice – you till the soil, you put the manure, you put an alphonso mango tree. You can't say you're 'mangoing.' You can't. You have to do the sadhana first. Can I sit for mango? Mango will happen if you do sadhana – if you do the practice of spiritual growth which is tilling the soil and giving the manure. Mango will happen as a result of your practice of spiritual growth. In the West, they have a lesser concept of what sadhana is. Sadhana is a continuous process of self-disciplined evolutionary action. Sadhana is sat-tat abhyas and sat-tat abhyas produces vairagya. So the fruit of vairagya will come through the repetitive practice of Kriya Yoga. It must be continuous, and it must be repetitive. And Kriya Yoga has that because Kriya Yoga is not for the lazy. And if you breath continuously, the laziness will also go.

So Kriya Yoga is a process of spinal breathing. It evolves your consciousness. It pierces the knots in your spine, which is called the shad-chakra bedhan. It is a very advanced sadhana which the Himalayan great masters have made simple for the grahasta to practice – it is for householders to practice. Kriya Yoga (ek sanjeev ni sadhana he) and you can conquer and overcome death like yogis of the Himalayas. And then there comes a time when you can say, "oh death, where is thy sting? Oh grave, where is thy victory?"

Whatever I say of Kriya Yoga is less and that's why it necessitated me to give you the experience to show you the difference. I'm not saying I'm inferior to others; I'm not saying I'm superior. I'm just saying I'm one of the few people who has given you the experience of Kriya Yoga – already given you anu graha on Kriya Yoga without you asking for it – so easily. Because my mandar is full – my mandar is Babaji. I've got zillions of dollars.

Gyanavatar Sri Yukteswar went and said in the West, "had India no other gift to offer to the world, Kriya Yoga and Raja Yoga would itself suffice as a kingly offering." These are the words of Gyanavatar Sri Yukteswar. This is very good, and I hope you take the most advantage.

I promise you that, if I am in America, and you call me and say, "Gurunath, there are forty people sitting in a circle, we've kept your asana here, can you give us a shakti-path?" from the United States of America, I will do it. Because I have the wherewithal. You have to go to the Guru who has the wherewithal. So, if I'm in Greenland or Europe or Italy or anywhere, if anything comes in the way of your Kriya Yoga, I'm prepared to remove it. But if you're not a spiritual practitioner towards God, I will first attend to the spiritual practitioners – those of you who are practising Kriya Yoga – then I'll see others who are not practising.

I wish to know; how do I find myself?

Kriya Yoga and Surya Yoga are the lightning path to finding your true self. What is preventing you finding your true self, or self-realization? This is what is preventing it – you put the hands of your mind upon the eyes of your soul and cry that you cannot see. Take away the hands of your mind from the eyes of your soul and behold the moon of your delight. Behold your true self. So, your mind is the obstruction. It is the dung of the mind which is covering the splendour of your soul. You all know how much nonsense you think in twenty-four hours and how much of real thoughts – real thoughts must be five or ten percent and nonsense must be ninety percent. That's how it is for human beings. But you are the valiant ones – you are the Vikram Adityas and Karnas and Arjunas who fight against ninety percent of your negativity and still you come out victorious on top. Give yourselves a hand.

So, in sadhana, what do you want? You want three things. Like when Narada came and said, "hey Rama, you are nothing, you are just a person. You may be Vishnu's avatar, but how can you compete with Ravana? Ravana is coming through the skies blazing in his chariot of fire with all of his armour and he is invincible. He cannot be killed." So, Rama told him, "hold on, don't get excited." He says, "there are a few qualities which will make me win. Discrimination and courage, these are my horses. My chariot is truth - satya. The wheels of my chariot are the powers of the Sun. I will be victorious. This is what Prabhu Ramchandra said."

This is a world of froth and bubbles – everyone is dancing to this facade. "In this world of froth and bubbles, two things stand alone – empathy in another's struggles and courage in your own." See, you must learn these things and when you be with people like me, I'm a madman. I'm courageous. So you'll also become a courageous madman. Because there's no sense in being cowardly – there's only one bullet in your name and when that bullet hits you, it has to hit you. You can die only once. Cowards may die many times, but the brave die only once, so be bold and live. Courage is the medicine. Courage is the balm, and I'm giving you the balsam. You have to have this.

You're living in the land of Goraksha. Lord Shiva himself incarnated on Earth as Shiva-Goraksha-Babaji. Do the mantra. Protect yourself against all ignorance, against premature death, and do the Surya.

I had downloaded some literature from the internet for aura purification wherein they talked about imagining the chakras like, say, Muladhara chakra is a red ball spinning clockwise, breath in red, breath out red. For other chakras various methods are given. So I would just like to understand from you how safe, unsafe, or beneficial these things would be.

You see, people talk a lot. Okay? So there's more of talk. It would be safe for the person who can throw his prana and breath through your breathing. If he can throw his prana and breath through your breathing, he can also control your chakras. I've got that technique in my God Healing 3 with mantras and chants – how to rotate the chakras; how to cure. But masters are few. If there are masters who can do the ayam (expansion and control) of prana, like what I did with you – I showed my prana with you to show you that you and I are one. So, all those guys come to me – all these great Reiki masters once came to me and the pranic healing master, he says, "I've got this thing here, can you heal me?" But he said, "don't tell anybody that you healed me, because I'm a great Reiki master." So, I healed them. Once I took a whole session of pranic healing masters – there were about a hundred people in there – and I healed them all together and I said, "a gift from me today, I'll heal you all."

Because these are small fragments of the real yoga I'm talking about –Kundalini Kriya Yoga and Patanjali's Raj Yoga, is the real yoga – and what you are telling me are just the fragments which are flying out. So I've done this many, many lives in the past. You come here, learn the simple Surya Yoga, and be happy. Don't complicate your mind with that too much. Don't distract your mind too much. Focus and don't fritter away the energies of your mind in a hundred-and-one things. Focus your mind. Collect your energies and focus on the Supreme. If you master one, you'll master everything. This is very, very important.

And another thing, for Bombay people, they say, "we have no time." Their watches are very dear and they're running on the clock, and that running on the clock has made them very, very time-bound. The demon time is killing them. The pace is killing the people before their time, bringing psychosomatic disorders. What I'm saying is that you will never get time to practise yoga and meditate on God - you have to make time.

Yogiraj Gurunath Siddhanath

Eliminate the I of Ego to See the Eye of the Soul

Each one must take personal responsibility for his own welfare. Humanity is endowed with a very delicate nervous system, brain structure, and astral system of chakras and the thousand-petal lotus. If he doesn't look after his delicate mechanism for the evolution of his own consciousness, then who will? The Sat – of the Sat-Chit-Ananda within you. God has given a spark of his within you and that's pushing from within without. It depends on the degree of your motivation – the inner push which will evolve you. If you choose to stay in slumber and darkness, then you shall. But the main courage of man, is that even in the darkness, he wants to see the light. And the light shineth in the darkness, and the darkness comprehended it not. The darkness can never comprehend the light, for the light is the dispeller of all darkness. Even a little bit of light can dispel the darkness of ignorance.

What sort of a learning do we have, its all-academic – we call this in English– if you try to get down to the details of what you are doing, it is called educare. You are being educated – education – because in Greek educare means "to bring in the light." How do your modern schools and systems educate you? They're just informing you. Your computers are good; your iPhones are better. I was very attracted to iPhone and I said it's a great toy because it's so good, you don't have to think. Everything is on the screen, there's no keyboard, nothing. But all the same, these things inform. They are information, but it's not education. It's not bringing in the light. You only get what you feed into the computer.

You see, you have to activate your own soul iPhone, and you can only activate your iPhone by seeing the eye (points at the third eye). To see the eye, you have to eliminate the bodily "I" – to see the eye of the soul, you must eliminate the I of the ego. So, to see the soul eye, you must eliminate the I, and then your iPhone (eye-Phone) will work. Your iPhones will not work till the I of the ego is a static and a way between your eye and I. But you must know which I/eye to eliminate and which I/eye to keep. What we're doing is we're keeping the wrong I/eye and therefore the true eye cannot be seen. Initially, it's very difficult to tell between a crystal and a diamond, but as you get practise with a trained eye, you shall be able to tell the diamond from the glass – the crystal glass. So you have to practise – be the diamond cutter of the diamond of your soul.

The seeing of the spiritual eye assumes prime importance in this time, where you can be steady and contact your intuition – get in touch with your conscience – and do what is truly right for you. There are no relative things like vice and virtue, good and bad, light and dark, and high and low, and personal ethics and global ethics. The only thing there is is before your eyes – don't complicate a simple thing by the spaghetti of your words and get stuck in the spaghetti of your words. A land yourself in a state of analysis paralysis. You can't do that – you have to be simple.

Your only object in this world is God and, knowing God, you'll know everything. All sufferings and the sufferings of others will be eliminated. You think God does not know what is happening in this world? It's all a screenplay on the screen of life. It's all a cosmic motion picture – a play of light and shadows – but we think that the light and shadows are true. Our mind is being deluded – we are mistaking the effect for the cause. We have to do the work given to us in this life, and that is to seek God in this life, in spite of all distractions. The only purpose of man's sojourn on this Earth is to seek God, period. Lecture over. This is it, long and short.

But then the mind is so fidgety and finicky and it's so intellectual in its tapestry that it wants to tap this, that, and the other, and have its finger in every pie. So, let's give the mind some exercise. The mind is like the monkey – you have to make him go up and down the pole of the spine until he gets exhausted by the practise of Kriya Yoga. Transform all your thoughts into the flaming star. That's the practise of Kriya Yoga – bind your mind to God and nothing else by Kriya Pranayama.

But how is that practical? Of course, it's the most practical thing, but it doesn't work according to our logic. God has his own logic – he has his own ways, and he will make it work. And even if he doesn't make it work, so what, God? I still love you. This is the brave soul. God, if you love me, I love you; if you kick me, I love you; if you praise me, I love you. I will love you whatever. This is my decision and I've made up my mind. Now you do what you want. Don't worry me and tempt me and harass me with these petty Ferraris and these little toys – I'm for God alone. Every breath belongs to You. And You are the one who tests us before putting us on the high seas.

He tests you with money, with name, with fame, and Ferraris, and whatever. So you have to see through this and know that the only purpose, the main purpose, the core purpose of your life is to progress towards your parent source and he is your parent source. You cannot help but gravitate towards him when Meditation deepens.

Yesterday, right before the satsang, for a period of fifteen seconds, I saw sparks just sparkling all around you like sparks coming out of a fire. Is that related to the sparks you were speaking of?

Yes, you can see it any time. Once I was in a company – a German company – and I was getting used to meditating long hours, but when I went to this temporary job of mine, I didn't get the time for meditation. So I went to the restroom, and I felt very peaceful there, and I just moved out of my body. Once I was trying very hard to meditate and get into that state – outer-body state – I couldn't get into that state. It was raining a lot, and at that time we were just beginning – about thirty to forty years back – we just started the yoga class and my class, it used to leak, so I used to close it in winter because we used to just take it in an old hall in Pune. Some of you have seen that place – you've come to my house. There used to be a huge puddle of water in the old hall. I didn't have the money and I was doing everything. That day, we had announced it's a class, so I came with a bucket and an old towel, and I was mopping it and sitting on my haunches and suddenly, I would ride out of my body. So, at certain stages he gives it to you when you least expect it. I had the samadhi experience

And this is the wealth – this is when God wants you to have it all. These people, the basic thing is, they are going into the objective sphere. It is the Western mind – it goes outward. The Indian mind is usually subjective – it goes inwards. He wants you to have the inner experience. If you have all the Ferraris, all the wealth in the world, all the wine, women, and laughter in the world, and your mind is in a depression or in sorrow, then you're in hell. If you're in the material heaven and your mind is a mess, then you're in hell. But if you're in actual hell and your mind is dancing with the light and love and power of God and his glory, then even in hell, you're in heaven. So, heaven and hell is not determined by the place – heaven and hell is determined by your inner state of consciousness. It's by your state of mind.

It's not the action which is a sin – it is the spirit in which it is done which makes it a vice or a virtue. The action itself is not a vice of a virtue. If, out of malice, I take a gun and shoot one person, it is a sin because the spirit is malice. If I take the same gun and turn around and fight for my country and shoot a hundred people, I get a medal of honor. Same gun, same man, but one is vice and one is virtue. What is this? Relativity of global ethics. One man's food is another man's poison. So the guy who is hailed as a great war hero in his own country may be the devil in the other country. That's why global ethics and personal ethics are relative terms. It can change – it depends on what your values are. Your values determine your ethics. Your soul essence determines your values.

Your global ethics may be to sit and direct contact with God; my global ethics may be just to keep building hospitals for the sick and the poor. And you cannot convince me that your merging into God in samadhi is in anyway better than my building hospitals for poor children. Although, as a matter of fact, I know of course merging into God in samadhi [is better], but that's Gurunath – the people will not know. I'm saying, just collecting pebbles by the riverside and with full faith offering them at the feet of the Lord, this is my devotion and there is nothing higher than that, and nobody in the world can convince me that [something else] is better than that. Or feeding children every Saturday – that's my religion, that's my prayer. I don't want your samadhi, I don't want your yoga, I don't want your high talk nor your high states. Just feeding children. So these are all relative terms. In relativity, there is no standardization of ethics. What is the global ethics? What is the standardization? It's all relative to one's personal karma.

I've heard that yogis – that practising Kriya Yoga take a long time, like a hundred years, to reverse the ageing process – so they're practising something else called Kaya Kalpa to keep the body young until the Kriya Yoga kicks in.

Your question is pretty mixed up I'll clear it. Firstly, the people who started the Kriya Yoga and the body immortality are a group of people called the Nath Yogis. I belong to the Nath tradition. There's a great misunderstanding. The body is the not-self. The spiritual soul is the True self. So why are you giving so much importance to body immortality over your own Divinity. First comes God, then comes body immortality. If you seek God in this life, there is no need to make your body immortal. The body immortality comes by His present grace judged by your past effort. This should be your attitude. This is the spiritual philosophy on which we stand. With this in mind, Nath Yogis practice body immortality to be Enlightened in the same body in the same life! In true yoga there is no place for the lazy. Divine grace is always won by sincere merit and devotional practice, called Sadhana and abyas.

We don't give body immortality priority over God like Leonard Orr did. Leonard Orr started a process of rebirthing and he reversed the process. He thought, "I had it." I also had a talk, like I had a talk with Yogi Bhajan, I met Haidakhan Baba. Haidakhan Baba is a great soul and I met him on more than one occasion. And I told him, "look, you have given this pranayama to the American people. They have somehow altered it – kept the idea of the yogic pranayama and they are using it for the primal scream and rebirthing. They are retrograding and going back to body consciousness instead of Divine Consciousness– a reversing-to-the-womb experience of a psychology." So then he said, "you're there – you go and correct it." So, I said, this is fine – this may be my work – and so for many years I was correcting the people who got stuck in their unfilming, going back to their negative subconscious mind, to the womb experience which they would have had at their time of birth. Why do you have to go back? Go forward. put on the light; the darkness will go. You have to evolve forward to the birth here (points to the third eye) – the Second Coming of the Christ is here. Third eye. The immaculate conception is here. This is important. The birth of the baby Krishna is in the third eye. You are born anew into the spiritual dimension of the Krishna Consciousness. This is what the true meaning of rebirthing and born anew is being from is being born into Divine Consciousness. Its called dvij the twice born.

The Time is Running Out

Let not precious moments slip by
Seek now the ultimate Truth.
Oh Thou Swan spread
Your wings to fly
Immortal realms
That death defy!

I said this poem to urge my disciples to move on! A famous poet has said that – most probably it is in the Rubaiyat.

> One moment in annihilation's waste,
> One moment of the well of life to taste,
> The stars are setting and the caravan
> Starts for the dawn of nothing,
> Oh make haste...

So, this dawn of nothing is not perceived by the Western mind. They want things: money, name, fame, Ferraris, friends, but they don't understand that "the stars are setting, and the caravan starts for the dawn of nothing, Oh, make haste." The dawn of nothing is God and he is indescribable, and therefore, he is called the dawn of nothing. "One moment in annihilation's waste, one moment of the well of life to taste, the stars are setting, and the caravan starts for the dawn of nothing, Oh, make haste." Don't keep sleeping and having me wake you up every morning. Don't miss the dawn of nothing, because the dawn of everything is beset with delusion, illusion, and error. It's only the purity of the dawn of nothing which will give you eternal bliss.

The idea is to touch some untouched corner of your heart and being, and awaken within you that nostalgic perfume which takes you to the land beyond description with joy ineffable. So most probably it is Khayyam who said this in one of his poems. Take care of your own karma, make your own formula, but do not forget the pathway to God. For he is the Truth, and ever shall be.

The Only Purpose of Our Sojourn on This Earth is To Seek God

I have many opportunities to act, to give, and to work. What guidance do you have between a global effort or a local effort? How does one find the good works?

Our first choice is God. We choose God first, and then other things of relativity. fastest way is by the practice of Kriya Yoga.

Now there are other choices which are secondary, compared to God – that choice you can make on your own. The prime purpose of man's sojourn on this Earth is to seek God. People doing anything else are delaying their evolution and enlightenment. Does this ring clear in your ears?

The second thing you can do is your bread-earning stuff. Put food on the table, okay? The third choice is whatever you want to do. You want to be working in Seaworld or Disneyland as a press reporter in the battle arena as a soldier in the army, that is your choice and it doesn't really matter. If there is a confusion in your mind, thank God: Don't do it. Practise Kriya Yoga. This is my simple way of thinking. But understand your professional calling shall be as per your past karma. Still do your Yoga as a lifestyle and evolve! To Reality in duality!

Create God within your being. He shall be a guiding light, He shall be your beacon: The beacon of Light shall guide you. Surrender to God first – Seek ye first the Kingdom of God, then all other problems shall be solved. And if they aren't, who cares?

> Oh Lord, as long as I have
> Thy Light before me, to guide me.
> And once I have Thee,
> I shall want no more.

I mean that's the sort of answer you'll expect from a yogi – any yogi. What else to you expect? We're here for God: Live God. Drink God. Be God. Love God. Be saturated with Him so much that when you explode with Him, you can explode with Love.

It appears that the good side is losing, with all these guys aggressing and terrorizing the earth. But I think if it is His wish and will, it will happen for a certain time – the cloud will pass, and there will be peace and good will on Earth. Let us see what happens. But practise Kriya Yoga with patience and I promise you that starting with you yourself, a lot of things will progress. You will not get what you want – you will get only what you need.

So, no ego-balm, no pampering, no gizmos. In the land of entertainment, you'll have to make a wee bit of sacrifice and lead the simple life, to get to the ordinary essence of life called Sahaj-Samadhi.

REALITY OF KRIYA YOGA
IS REVELATION OF
THE REALITY ITSELF!

Appendix

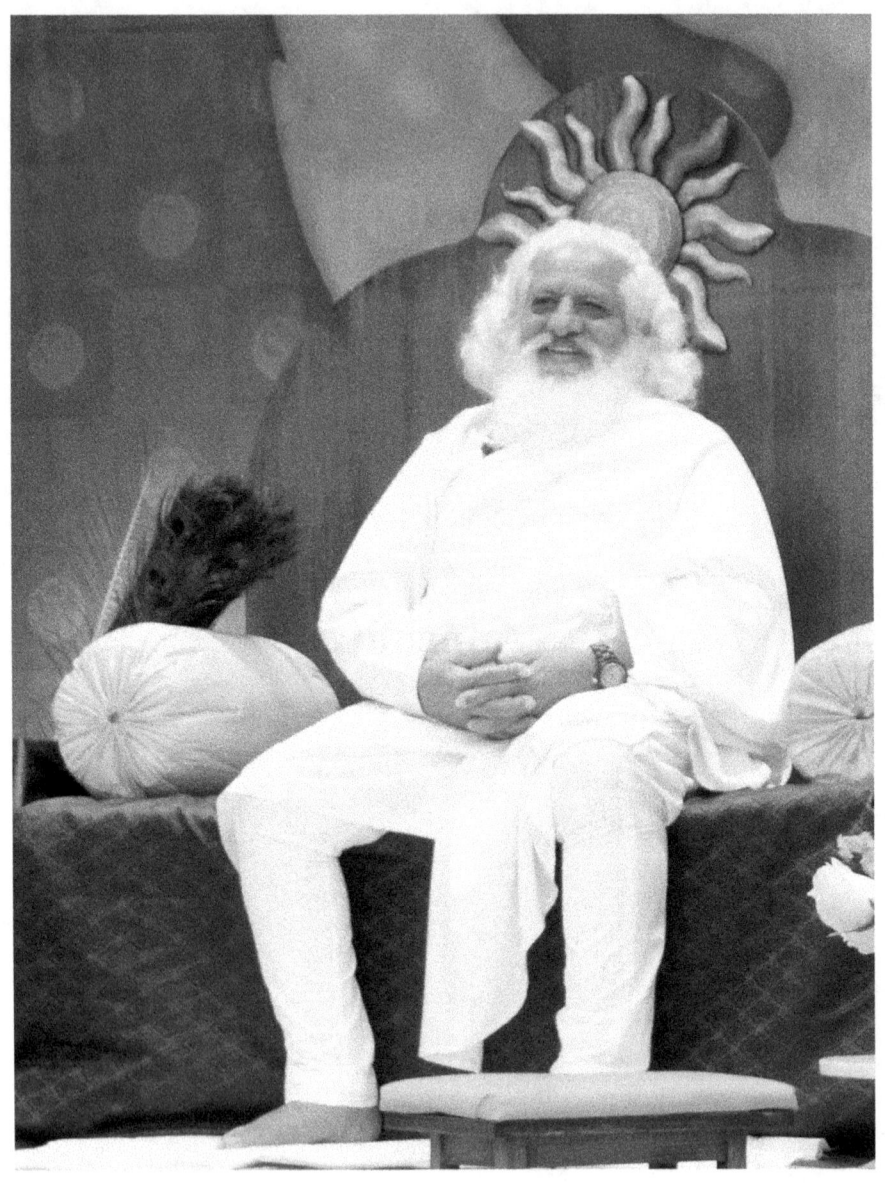

Yogiraj SatGurunath Siddhanath

A brief introduction to his teachings

His Life

Yogiraj Sat Gurunath was born on May 10th, 1944. He is a Siddha by birth and belongs to one of the premier families of Gwalior, India. Educated in Sherwood College [Nainital], he spent his early years in the Himalayas with the great Nath Yogis, in whose presence he was transformed. The Divine Transformation was completed by his deep and personal experience with Mahavtar Babaji (Shiva-Goraksha-Nath Babaji) – the same immortal introduced by Yogananda in his classic, 'Autobiography of a Yogi'. Yogiraj is a direct disciple of Babaji and with his blessings has founded the Siddhanath Yoga Parampara.

Yogiraj now teaches various ancient forms of Yoga founded by the Nath Tradition, such as Mahavatar Babaji Kriya Yoga. He bestows powerful Shaktipat transmissions and unique 'Thought Free' Sates of Raja Yoga which empower the practitioners to gradually go into Samadhi (awareness of one's own Self), experiencing the depths of Eternal Being. Lord Krishna's vision has given him to realize the oneness of all yogas, faiths and religions.

His Genius

Besides the Himalayan Masters, SatGurunath is the only Siddha known to us and broadly accessible, who gives authentic experiences of Shaktipat Kundalini Energy Transmission created specifically for spiritual and healing transformation essential to the awakening and continued evolution of humankind. The sincere will receive these dimensions of the Guru's consciousness through direct experience as to what true yoga is rather than through intellectual exploration.

The Reality of Kriya Yoga

The experience of SatGurunath's Consciousness will be bestowed as the Guru guides the seeker in transforming his thought-filled finite mind into infinite consciousness free of thoughts.

Herein lies the Genius of Gurunath - with a flash he bestows upon you His Consciousness of Natural Enlightenment, transforming the ripples of thought in your mind's lake into a waveless lake of Soul Awareness bereft of thought. With flawless clarity during this passage he keeps intact the awareness of ones individual self as the boundaries of it's I-ness melt into the knowing of one's own boundless Awareness. This process he calls "Shivapat".

The mind's I-ness will resist its soul consciousness expanding into super consciousness out of fear of losing its ego identity. But this is not the truth. The complete truth is that the individual mind loses its identity only to partake its vaster identity as infinite awareness, the drop merges into the ocean not to lose itself but to become of it.

Panapat is the Uniqueness of Gurunath where with utter simplicity by breathing through us he brings to you Shiv Goraksha Babaji's Kriya Yoga and the Timeless Yoga of the Nath Yogis. He has simplified the arduous Nath techniques, yet preserved the effectiveness of the sacred practices. As a living master, he offers to humanity his own clear-mind consciousness. In sharing this experience with each individual seeker personally and with thousands of receptive people the world over simultaneously, Sat Gurunath as "The Presence" reveals the secret that at the level of pure consciousness all Humanity is One.

The Nath Lineage of Kriya Yoga

As we peer into the akashic records of the misty past we get a glimpse of the lineage of the Nath Yogis. It began from Adi Nath, Lord Shiva Himself, who gave it to His consort Parvati, Uday Nath. She gave it to Vishnu - Santosh Nath, Ganesh and Nandi Nath. Then Lord Krishna as Vishnu initiated Lord Vivasvat, the Spirit of our

Sun. The lineage was later guarded by the Kings of the Solar Dynasty: Vaivasvat Manu, King Ikshavaku down to Harishchandra, then to Lord Raghu Nath (Rama), 47th in descent from Ikshavaku. He is the 8th Rudra, esoterically connected with Shiv Goraksha Babaji, who is an incarnation of Lord Shiva Himself. It is through this grand lineage of the Nath Yogis that the royal science of Kriya Yoga has been preserved and handed down through the corridors of time by the ever-living Shiva- Goraksha-Babaji. It is to this lineage that Yogiraj Gurunath belongs – blessed by Babaji to spread this divine science in the East and West.

His Hallmark : The Knowing of a True Master

A Satguru or Empowering Master can be known by three distinct graces he bestows upon his disciples.
- Transmit – center to center in their pranic chakras – the evolutionary Kundalini Energy: **Shaktipat**
- Breathe the powerful breath through the breathing of disciples in their Spinal channels: **Pranapat**
- Impart his consciousness of thought free enlightenment to the receptive: **Shivapat**

Only a Master who showers all three blessings on truth seekers is a true Satguru. Gurunath bestows all three blessings.

Wings to Freedom – The Journey of the Soul

The way of the white swan is the evolution of human consciousness, the most comprehensive enterprise ever undertaken by humanity, besides which the greatest of human achievements pale into insignificance. This process is Yoga, which commends itself to the foremost minds of East and West. In the human brain exists the lateral ventricles in the shape of a "Swan in Flight" with its head pointing to the back as though the swan is flying faster than light back to the future. When the Hamsa Yogi, through meditation and pranayam, activates the Kundalini energy, then these ventricles in the brain open up. The two petals in the Agya Chakra, corresponding to the pituitary gland, open. The Yogi, at this stage, experiences Hamsa Consciousness, being breathed by the Divine Indweller.

The Sushumna channel in the spinal chord is the highway through which the Kundalini Energy travels and the evolution of consciousness takes place. It is the kinetic energy remaining after the completion of the universe. This force lies as light/sound vibrations potentially coiled around the swayambhu linga in the mooladhar chakra. To avail of it for one's own evolution and realization is the birthright of every human soul. It may be awakened by yogic procedures - best by Unmani, a no-mind state of absorption.

As the Hamsa Nath Yogi progresses in the Hamsa meditation, the third eye opens up in the Agya Chakra and he goes into the Sarvikalpa consciousness. Then, by further practice, he penetrates the Star of the Eye and expands to the Paramahamsa Nath Yogi state of Nirvikalpa consciousness, dwelling in the Cave of Brahma , the brain's third ventricle. Then his awareness evolves further beyond the I-ness of humanity to settle in the lateral swan-like ventricles of the brain, where he becomes the Siddha Nath Yogi. The mighty Hamsa soul has won its wings to freedom. As the subtle fibers of the Corona Radiata light up with Divine effulgence he takes flight into Cosmic consciousness as the Avadhoot Nath Yogi. He experiences the total Divinity of and beyond creation, gaining the ultimate knowledge of "Tat Tvam Asi" - "That Thou Art". The Yogi then merges into Niranjan, the final Nirvana, having attained the enlightenment of Buddha and Christ. This Avadhoot Nath Yogi returns to the world no more. If, under rare circumstances, he ever does, it will be the descent of Divinity as Avatar Nath Yogi.

SatGurunath's Vision for World Peace
Hear Our Soul Call!

If World Peace is to Herald the Dawn of a New Age, realize that
Humanity Our Uniting Religion
Breath Our Uniting Prayer and
Consciousness Our Uniting God

Glossary

A

Abhyasa — practice, specifically of yoga

Acharya — a preceptor, instructor or teacher-guru

Adinath ("primordial Lord") — the founder of the Nath yogis, Shiva Himself

Advaita ("nonduality") — the truth and teaching that there is only One Reality called Atman or Brahman, especially as found in the Upanishads; see also Vedanta

Agya chakra (Center of Divine Presence) — a yogic appellation for the third eye center; also called ajna chakra

Ahamkara ("I-maker") — the individuation principle, or ego, which must be transcended; cf. asmitâ; see also buddhi, manas

Ahibudnya ("Unfathomable Serpent of the Deep") — an epithet of Shiva.

Ahimsa ("non-harming") — an important moral discipline (yama)

Aja (also aja ekapada) – ("the unborn"), a term used for the primordial Divine as well as its universal energy called Kundalini. As aja ekapada ("the unborn one-footed") Gurunath explains, "He who stands alone on one leg, without support."

Akasha ("ether/space") — the first of the five Cosmic elements of which the physical universe is composed; also used to designate "inner" space, that is, the space of consciousness (called cid-âkâsha)

Alakh Niranjana ("come great void") — a saying, greeting, and blessing voiced by Nath yogis

Amba ("darkness") — the "Great Deep", appellation for an aspect of the Divine Mother

Amrita ("immortal/immortality") — a designation of the deathless Soul (atman, purusha); also the nectar of immortality that flows from the psycho-energetic center at the crown of the head (see sahasrara-chakra) when it is activated and transforms the body into a "Divine body" (divya-deha)

Anahata (anahata-chakra) – ("wheel of the unstruck sound"), the twelve-petal lotus of the heart. The heart has since ancient times been viewed as the secret seat of the Divine and the location where

the immortal sound om can be heard. Its seed syllable (bija mantra) is yam pertaining to the element of wind.
Ananda ("bliss") — the condition of utter joy, which is an essential quality of the ultimate reality (tattva)
Ananda Kanda – below the twelve-petal anahata-chakra and within it is an eight-petal lotus, which is the seat of bliss called ananda kanda. It is located within the causal body, the anandamayeekosha (ananda- maya-kosha).
Anga ("limb") — a fundamental category of the yogic path, such as yama, niyama, asana, dharanâ, dhyana, pranayama, pratyahâra, samadhi
Annamayeekosha (anna-maya-kosha) – ("sheath composed of food"), the lowest of the five "envelopes" (kosha) covering the Self; the physical body
Apana – an aspect of the life-force energy functioning in the body for the purpose of excretion and elimination
Aranyaka ("that which pertains to the forest") — an early type of ritual text used by forest-dwelling sages; cf. Upanishad
Arbandha-Nag Langot — the wollen belts tied around the waist of the Nath Yogi extending to form a aprt of his under-garment; also calld the bhairava bana
Arti — the blessing of the light and sound during Divine worship
Arjuna ("White") — one of the five Pandava princes who fought in the "great war" depicted in the Mahabharata; disciple of the Avatar Krsna whose teachings can be found in the Bhagavad-Gita
Asana ("seat") — a physical posture (see also anga, mudra); the third limb (anga) of Patanjali's eightfold path (astha-anga-yoga); originally this meant only meditation posture, but subsequently, in Hatha Yoga, this aspect of the yogic path was developed further
Ashram ("that where effort is made") — a hermitage; also a stage of life, such as brahmacharya, householder, forest dweller, and complete renouncer (samnyasin)
Ashta-anga-yoga, ashtanga-yoga ("eight-limbed union") —the eightfold Yoga of Patanjali, consisting of moral discipline (yama), self-restraint (niyama), posture (asana), breath control (pranayama), sensory withdrawal (pratyahara), concentration (dharana), meditation (dhyana), and ecstasy (samadhi), leading to liberation (kaivalya)

Asmita ("I-am-ness") — a concept of Patanjali's eight-limbed Yoga, roughly synonymous with ahamkara

Atman ("self") — the true Self, or Spirit, which is eternal and Super- conscious; our true nature or identity; sometimes a distinction is made between the atman as the individual self and the parama-atman as the transcendental Self; see also purusha; cf. brahman

Aunsch Avatara – A partial Avatara that manifests only the degree of Divinity necessary to fulfill a specific mission

Aulia – a mad hermit

Avadhoot ("he who has shed everything") — a Nath Yogi who has gone through the 6th stage of initiation; by his effort and Divine grace, achieved the Divine Consciousness of the Avatar

Avasta ("condition") — the super-conscious states of yogic realization; different states are distinguished according to the stage of realization

Avatar ("descent") — a manifestation or incarnation of the Divine on earth; famous Avatars of the past are Rama, Krsna, and Buddha

Avidya ("ignorance") — the root cause of suffering (duhkha); also called ajnana; cf. vidya

Ayurveda ("life science") — one of India's traditional systems of medicine. The eldest of the world's medical systems. The Veda that prolongs life.

B

Babaji ("revered one") — specifically in the Nath tradition to denote the "Ancient of Days;" "The youth of 16 summers;" the ever-youthful immortal yogi, also mentioned in Yogananda's book, "Autobiography of a Yogi"

Bandha ("bond/bondage") — the fact that human beings are typically bound by ignorance (avidya), which causes them to lead a life governed by the law of karma rather than inner freedom generated through wisdom (vidya, jnana)

Bhagavad-Gita("Lord's Song") — the most popular book on the science of Yoga, embedded in the epic Mahabharata and containing the teachings of Karma Yoga (the path of self-transcending action), Jnana Yoga (the path of wisdom), and Bhakti Yoga (the path of devotion), and Raja Yoga (the supreme path of meditation) as given by the Avatar Krsna to Prince Arjuna on the battlefield of Kurushetra

Bhajan – from the word bhanjan "to divide;" devotional song whence the devotee is separate from Deity and does not fuse with God as does the yogi in samadhi

Bhakta ("devotee") — a disciple practicing Bhakti Yoga

Bhakti ("devotion/love") — the love of the bhakta toward the Divine or the Guru as a manifestation of the Divine

Bhakti Sutra ("Aphorisms on Devotion") — an aphoristic work on devotional Yoga authored by Sage Narada

Bhakti Yoga ("Yoga of devotion") — a major branch of the Yoga tradition, utilizing the feeling capacity to connect with the ultimate reality conceived as a personal Divinity

Bharat ("the land of India") — The land whose people are wedded to the light of the Soul.

Bija-mantra (Beej-mantra) – ("seed word"); a monosyllabic mantra, each of which is associated with one of the seven chakras of the body

Bindu ("seed/point") — the creative potency of anything where all energies are focused; the dot (also called tilaka) worn on the forehead as indicative of the third eye

Bodhi ("enlightenment") — the state of the awakened Master, or buddha

Bodhisattva ("enlightenment being") — in Mahayana Buddhist Yoga, the individual who, motivated by compassion (karuna), is committed to achieving enlightenment for the sake of all other beings

Brahma ("he who has grown expansive") — the Creator of the universe, the first principle (tattva) to emerge out of the ultimate reality (brahman)

Brahma Gufa — see Cave of Brahma

Brahmacharya — (from brahma and charya "brahmic conduct") the discipline of chastity, which produces ojas

Brahman ("that which has grown expansive") — the ultimate reality (cf. âtman, purusha)

Buddha ("awakened") — a designation of the person who has attained enlightenment (bodhi) and therefore inner freedom; term designating Gautama, the founder of Buddhism, who lived in the sixth century BCE

Buddhi ("that which is conscious, awake") — the higher mind, which is the seat of wisdom (vidya, jnana); cf. manas

Bhuta ("to become") — the material elements, also called pancha bhuta, or five elements of earth (prithvi), water (apas), fire (agni), air (vata), and space (akasha)

Bhuta Shuddhi ("purification of the elements") — transformation of the gross physical body into a Divine body, by dissolving the five elements

C

Cave of Brahma ("Brahma Gumfa") — the brain's third ventricle; a hollow space in the human brain formed by the thalimus as its walls, the hypothalimus as its floor, and the third choroid plexus as its roof

Chakra ("pranic wheel") — the psycho-energetic centers of the subtle body (sukshma-sharir). Classically seven of such centers are given: muladhara chakra at the perineum, svadhishthana chakra at the base of the spine, manipura chakra at the navel, anahata chakra at the heart, vishuddhi chakra at the throat, ajna chakra in the middle of the head, and sahasrara chakra at the top of the head

Cit ("consciousness") — the super-conscious ultimate reality (see Atman, Brahman, Chaitanya)

Citta ("mind-substance") — ordinary consciousness, the mind, as opposed to cit

Citi ("shakti") — the kinetic energy shakti; cf. kundalini

D

Dakini — a sky-walker; a semi-divine female being, sometimes progressing one's spiritual practice and sometimes obstructing it.

Darshana ("vision" or "sight") — vision in the literal and spiritual sense; a system of philosophy, such as the yoga-darshana of Patanjali

Deva ("he who is shining") — a male deity, such as Shiva, Vishnu, or Brahma, either in the sense of the ultimate reality or a high angelic being

Devi ("she who is shining") — a female deity such as Pârvatî, Lakshmî, or Saraswati, either in the sense of the ultimate reality (in its feminine aspect) or a high angelic being

Dhaba – India roadside food well cooked

Dharana ("holding") — concentration, the sixth limb (anga) of Patanjali's eight-limbed Yoga

Dharma ("bearer") — a term of numerous meanings; often used in the sense of "law," "lawfulness," "virtue," "righteousness," "norm"

Dhuni — the sacred fires of the ancient yogis, which they revere as holy and sustain themselves for cooking and warmth. Dhunis leave behind gow-rakh, alkaline cow dung ash that the yogis smear on their body in order to prevent disease.

Dhyana ("ideating") — meditation, the seventh limb (anga) of Patanjali's eight-limbed Yoga

Diksha ("initiation") — the act and condition of induction into the hidden aspects of Yoga or a particular lineage of teachers; all traditional Yoga is initiatory

Divya-deha (also Divya-vapus) – ("Divine body"), a Divine body of radiant light created by yogic ingestion of mercury, pranayama, diet, and God's grace. An immaculate body of rainbow light, free from the ravages of time for the purpose of uninterrupted communion with God.

Divya Guru ("Divine preceptor") — a Sat-Guru who works from a higher plane of existence

Duhkha ("bad axle space") — suffering, a fundamental fact of life, caused by ignorance (avidya) of our true nature (the Self or atman)

G

Gandha – A smell, aroma

Gayatri mantra — a famous Vedic mantra recited particularly at sunrise

Ghagara-chunari – A style of dress in Rajasthan and Northern India including a tunic, top, and shawl.

Ghat — a small temple in Banares along the holy river Ganges for worship and bathing rituals; an honor granted only to certain select families

Gheranda-Samhita("Sage Gheranda's Compendium") — one of three major manuals of classical Hatha Yoga, composed in the seventeenth century; cf. Hatha-Yoga-Pradipika, Shiva-Samhita

Goraksha ("Cow Protector") — the immortal (also called Babaji, Gorakshanath, and Shiva-Goraksha-Babaji) traditionally said to be the founding adept of Hatha Yoga, a disciple of Matsyendranath

Gorakshanath ("lord Goraksha") — the most documented and recent appearance of Shiva-Goraksha-Babaji, to speed the spiritual evolution of humanity. The personal aspect of Lord Shiva.

Goshti — spiritual chat from a Guru

Gotri — spiritual lineage

Granthi ("knot") — any one of three common blockages in the central pathway (sushumna-nadi) preventing the full ascent of the serpent power (kundalini-shakti); the three knots are known as brahma granthi (at the muladhara chakra), the Vishnu granthi (at the heart), and the rudra granthi (at the third-eye center)

Guna ("quality") — refers to any of the three primary "qualities" or constituents of nature (prakriti): tamas (the principle of inertia), rajas (the dynamic activity), and sattva (the principle of luminosity)

Guru ("one with gravity") — a teacher who cultivates the spiritual knowledge of a disciple

Guru-bhakti ("teacher devotion") — a disciple's self-transcending devotion to the guru; see also bhakti

Guru-Yoga ("Yoga (relating to) the teacher") — a yogic approach that makes the Guru the center of a disciple's practice; all traditional forms of Yoga contain a strong element of Guru-yoga

H

Hamsa ("swan") — the Soul, the individuated Consciousness (jiva); also refers to the life-breath (prana) as it moves within the body; the lateral ventricles in the human brain in the shape of a swan in flight, with its wings thrust toward the forehead and its posterior ventricle pointed to the back, like a swan flying back to the future, faster than light; see jiva-atman; see also param-hamsa

Hamsacharya — a teacher of the Hamsa Yoga Sangh; an adept of the 2nd level of initiation

Hamsakriyacharya — an adept of the 3rd level of initiation Hamsanet – Yogiraj Gurunath's personal work; the astral light connection between all Gurunath's disciples (Hamsas) with the Guru and to one another

Hatha Yoga ("Forceful Yoga") — a major branch of Yoga, developed by Gorakshanath and his disciples c. 1000CE, and emphasizing the physical aspects of the transformative path, notably postures (asana) and cleansing techniques (shodhana), but chiefly breath control (pranayama)

Hatha-Yoga-Pradipika ("Light on Hatha-Yoga") — one of three classical manuscripts on Hatha Yoga, compiled by Svatmarama in the fourteenth century

Hiranyaloka ("golden world") — the highest astral heaven of luminosity to which some yogis ascend, to practice higher forms of Yoga under the guidance of Divine Teachers (Divya Gurus) such as Shri Yukteswar

I

Ida nadi ("pale conduit") — the prana current or arc ascending on the left side of the central channel (sushumna-nadi) associated with the parasympathetic nervous system and having a cooling or calming effect on the mind when activated; cf. pingala-nadi

Indriya ("concerning Indra") — refers to the five senses of sight, hearing, taste, smell, touch, and the corresponding organs of sense

Ishta Devata – The principle aspect of God according to one's devotion

Ishvara ("ruler") — the Lord; referring either to the Creator (see Brahma) or, in Patanjali's yoga-darshana, to a special transcendental Self (purusha)

Ishvara-pranidhana ("dedication to the Lord") — surrender to the Lord; in Patanjali's eight-limbed Yoga one of the practices of self-restraint (niyama); see also Bhakti-Yoga

Ishwara-Sanatana – ("God Eternal"), the Mahavatara, Shiva-Goraksha-Babaji

J

Jain — pertaining to the jinas ("conquerors"), the liberated adepts of Jainism; a member of Jainism, the spiritual tradition founded by Mahavira, a contemporary of Gautama the Buddha

Japa ("muttering") — the repeated recitation of mantras

Jivatman or Jiva ("individual self") — the individuated consciousness, as opposed to the ultimate Self (parama atman)

Jivanmukta ("he who is liberated while alive") — an adept who, while still embodied, has attained liberation (moksha)

Jivanmukti ("living liberation") — the state of liberation while being embodied

Jnana ("knowledge/wisdom") — both worldly knowledge or world-transcending wisdom, depending on the context; see also prajna; cf. vidyâ

Jnana Yoga ("Yoga of wisdom") — the path to liberation based on wisdom, or the direct intuition of the transcendental Self (atman) through the steady application of discernment between the real and the unreal and renunciation of what has been identified as unreal (or inconsequential to the achievement of liberation)

K

Kaivalya ("isolation") — the state of absolute freedom from conditioned existence, as explained in Ashtanga Yoga; in the non-dualistic (advaita) traditions of India, this is usually called moksha or mukti (meaning "release" from the fetters of ignorance, or avidya)

Kali — a Goddess embodying the fierce (dissolving) aspect of the Divine

Kali-yuga — the dark age of spiritual and moral decline, said to be current now; kali does not refer to the Goddess Kali but to the losing throw of a die

Kama ("desire") — the appetite for sensual pleasure blocking the path to true bliss (ananda); the only desire conducive to freedom is the impulse toward liberation

Kapila ("He who is red") — a great sage founder of the Samkhya tradition, who is said to have composed the Samkhya Sutra

Kara Hati – ("to do with the hands"); later known as the martial arts form, Karate.

Karma ("action") — activity of any kind, including ritual acts; said to be binding only so long as engaged in a self-centered way; destiny; law of cause and effect; the genetic code and social condition of an individual birth

Karma Yoga ("Yoga of action") — the liberating path of self- transcending action

Karmandalu — a pot made of copper and brass and used by yogis for carrying water.

Karuna ("compassion") —universal sympathy complementary to wisdom (prajnâ)

Kaulism (Kaula-marga) – The Kaul Tantra originated by Matsyendranatha as disclosed in the Kaula-Jnana-Nirnaya involving the Divinization of the body through stimulating the flow of "the nectar of immortality" (amrit)

Khecari mudra ("space-walking seal") — the yogic practice of curling the tongue back against the upper palate in order to seal the life energy (prana); also the piercing effect of the tongue when it can reach beyond the ulvula, stimulating the pituitary gland to drink of nectar.

Kosha ("casing") — any one of five "envelopes" surrounding the transcendental Self (atman) and thus blocking its light: annamaya-kosha ("envelope made of food," the physical body), pranamayakosha ("envelope made of life force"), manomaya-kosha ("envelope made of mind"), vijnanamaya-kosha ("envelope made of consciousness"), and anandamayakosha ("envelope made of bliss")

Krsna ("Puller") — an incarnation of God Vishnu, the Purna Avatar whose teachings can be found in the Bhagavad-Gita and the Bhagavata-Purana

Kriya Yoga ("Yoga of action with awareness") — the yogic path initiated by Babaji to speed up spiritual evolution

Kumbhaka ("potlike") — breath retention; cf. pûraka, recaka

Kundalini ("coiled spiral") — electro-magnetic pranic energy; kundalini is the lady of the cinders whom, when fanned by the alchemical fire of Shiva-shakti pranayam, ignites and blazes up the chimney of the spine to unite with the immortal Lord Shiva in the crown chakra (sahasrara) to enlighten the yogi.

Kundalin Kriya Yoga — when the Kriya Yoga pranayam is performed, the pranic life-force in one's spinal chord (sushumna) builds up to generate a great spiritual magnetism and voltage. By the ceaseles movement of the Kriya life-force, one's prana, breath, vital fluid, and mind become one to form the evolutionary life-force energy called Kundalini.

L

Lakulish ("the staff-holder") — He who holds the lightning-staff of evolution, a representation of Lord Shiva or Babaji-Gorakhnath. He si also deified as the ancient founder of the Shiva Pashupat sect of yogis.

Lateral Ventricles — When the consciousness of a yogi fills the lateral ventricles, he sees the hollow space in the form of a swan in flight with its wings thrust towards the forehead and its head pointing to the back as though the Soul Swan is flying back to the future faster than light; see Hamsa Swan

Laya Yoga ("Yoga of dissolution") — an advanced form or process of Tantric Yoga by which the energies associated with the various psycho-energetic centers (chakras) of the subtle body are gradually dissolved through the ascent of the serpent power (kundalini shakti)

Linga ("mark") — the pillar as a principle of creativity; a symbol of Shiva; a symbol for the universe cf. yoni

Lungi — A type of wraparound worn by the men of India

M

Mahabharata ("Great Bharata") — one of India's two great ancient epics telling of the great war between the Pandavas and the Kauravas and serving as a repository for many spiritual and moral teachings

Mahatma (from maha-atman, "great self") — an honorific title (meaning something like "a great soul") bestowed on particularly meritorious individuals, such as Gandhi

Manas ("mind") — the lower mind, which is bound to the senses and yields information (vijnana) rather than wisdom (jnana, vidya); cf. buddhi

Mandala ("circle") — a circular design symbolizing the cosmos and specific to a deity

Mantra (from the verbal root man "to think") — a sacred sound or phrase, such as om, hum, or om namah shivaya, that has a transformative effect on the mind of the individual reciting it; to be ultimately effective, a mantra needs to be given in an initiation by a Master

Mantra Yoga — the yogic path utilizing mantras as the primary means of liberation

Marman ("lethal spot") — in Ayurveda and Yoga, a vital spot on the physical body where energy is concentrated or blocked; cf. granthi

Matsyendranath ("Lord of Fish") — an early Nath and Mahasiddha, who founded the Yogini-Kaula school of Tantra and who implored Shiva to give him a disciple more advanced then himself; Shiva Himself came as Gorakshanath

Maya ("she who measures") — the deluding or illusive power of the world; illusion by which the world is seen as separate from the ultimate singular reality (atman)

Moksha ("release") — the condition of freedom from ignorance (avidya) and the binding effect of karma; also called mukti, kaivalya

Morchal — A fan made of peacock feathers for cleansing one's astral body and driving away negative forces

Mudra ("seal") — a hand gesture (such as chin mudra) or whole-body gesture (such as viparita karani mudra)

Mula-mantra ("root mantra") — the root mantra of a specific deity; in the case of Shiva, Om Namah Sivaya; in the case of Visnu, Om Namo Bagavate Vasudevaya

Muni ("he who is silent") — a silent sage

N

Nada ("sound") — the inner sound, as it can be heard through the practice of Nada Yoga or Kundalini Yoga

Nada Yoga ("Yoga of the inner sound") — the yoga or process of producing and intently listening to the inner sound as a means of concentration and ecstatic self-transcendence

Nadi ("conduit") — one of 72,000 subtle-astral channels along or through which the life force (prana) circulates; the three most important ones are the ida nadi, pingala nadi, and sushumna nadi

Nadi-shodhana ("channel cleansing") — the practice of purifying the conduits, especially by means of breath control (pranayama)

Narada — a great devotee of Shiva; a great sage associated with music, who taught Bhakti Yoga and is attributed with the authorship of one of two Bhakti-Sutras

Nath ("lord") — appellation for the greatest of yogic Masters, the Lords of all forms of Yoga; in particular adepts of the Kanphata ("Split- ear") school founded by Gorakshanath

Nath mandala — The electromagnetic spiritual field of the Nath Yogis Nava-Nath — The primeval Nine Naths of the seventh degree of cosmic awareness and beyond

Niranjana — highest state of consciousness or form of samadhi for the Naths

Nirbija — consciousness without seed; the higher forms of samadhi

Nirodha ("restriction") — in Patanjali's eight-limbed Yoga, the very basis of the process of concentration, meditation, and ecstasy; in the first instance, the restriction of the "whirls of the mind" (chitta-vritti)

Niyama ("self-restraint") — the second limb of Patanjali's eightfold path, which consists of purity (shauca), contentment (samtosha), austerity (tapas), study (svadhyaya), and surrender to the Lord (ishvara-pranidhana)

O

Ojas ("vitality") — the subtle energy produced through practice, especially the discipline of chastity (brahmacharya)

Om — the original mantra symbolizing the ultimate reality, which is prefixed to many mantric utterances; the ever-sounding hum of creation

Ot-prot Surya — ("Solar osmosis"); process of solar pranayam originated by Yogiraj Gurunath whereby the energy of the sun is inhaled and negativity is exhaled

P

Paramatman ("Supreme Self") — the transcendental Self, which is singular, as opposed to the individuated self (jiva-atman) that exists in countless numbers in the form of living beings

Paramahansa ("Supreme Swan") — the 4th level of initiation; an honorific title given to great adepts, such as Ramakrishna and Yogananda

Paramartha Satya – The Absolute Divine Truth, Bramha Nirvana

Parinam – ("transformation"); a term in Patanjali's Yoga Sutras denoting the serial transmutation of Consciousness; transmutation is not transformation but a sequential moving expansion of Consciousness as it ascends from grosser to subtler dimensions of mind

Patanjali — the great Siddha or perfected Master of Yoga who authored the Yoga-Sûtra.

Pingala-nadi ("reddish conduit") — the prana current ascending on the right side of the central channel (sushuma-nadi) and associated with the sympathetic nervous system and having an energizing effect on the mind when activated; cf. ida nadi

Prajna ("wisdom") — the opposite of spiritual ignorance (ajnana, avidya)

Prakriti ("creatrix") — nature, which is multilevel and, according to Patanjali's yoga-darshana, consists of an eternal dimension (called pradhana or "foundation"), levels of subtle existence (called sukshma- parvan), and the physical or coarse realm (called sthyla-parvan); all of nature is deemed unconscious (acit), and therefore it is viewed as being in opposition to the transcendental Self or Spirit (purusha)

Prana ("life"; "breathing forth") — the universal life-force enrgy animating the whole of creation, the breath of the Cosmic Parusha; in the individual, the vitality imparting Consciousness to sentient beings.

Pranapat — a term coined by Yogiraj Gurunath Siddhanath to denote the grace of a Sat-Guru, when he breathes through the breath of the disciple; cf shaktipat; shivapat

Pranayama (from prâna and âyâma, "life/breath extension") — breath control and expansion, the fourth limb (anga) of Patanjali's eightfold path, consisting of conscious inhalation (puraka), retention (kumbhaka), and exhalation (rechaka); at an advanced state, breath retention occurs spontaneously and for prolonged periods of time

Prasada ("grace/clarity") — Divine grace, mental clarity; food consecrated by the Guru or a deity.

Pratyahara ("withdrawal") — sensory inhibition, the fifth limb (anga) of Patanjali's eightfold path

Puja ("worship") — prescribed rituals usually accompanied by the recitation of mantras or shlokas, an important aspect of many forms of Yoga, notably Karma and Bhakti Yoga

Pujari (Pujarin) — The person who performs a puja, usually the temple Brahmin

Puraka ("filling in") — inhalation, an aspect of breath control (pranayama)

Purana ("Ancient") — often refering to the ancient spiritual literature of India dealing with royal genealogy, cosmology, philosophy, and ritual; there are eighteen major and many more minor works of this nature

Purusha ("male") — the transcendental Self (atman) or Spirit, a designation that is mostly used in Samkhya and Patanjali's yoga-darshana

R

Radha — the Avatar Krsna's spouse; a name of the Divine Mother

Raja Yoga ("Royal Yoga") — a late medieval designation of Patanjali's eightfold yoga-darshana, also known as Classical Yoga

Rama — an Avatar of Vishnu preceding Krsna; the principal hero of the Ramayana

Ramayana ("Rama's life") — one of India's two great national epics telling the story of Rama; cf. Mahâbhârata

Rechaka ("expulsion") — exhalation, an aspect of breath control (pranayama)

Reincarnation (Punar Janma) — the individual Soul rotating in the repeatd cycle of birth, death (the kala chakra) owing to bondage creating karma.

Rig-Veda — the most ancient literature and knowledge passed down from pre-history; see Veda

Rishi ("seer") — the Sages of Fire Mist; a category of Vedic sage; an honorific title of certain venerated masters and Cosmic Beings

S

Sadhana ("accomplishing") — spiritual discipline leading to siddhi ("perfection" or "accomplishment")

Sahaja ("together-born") — natural enlightenment; the fact that the transcendental reality and the empirical reality are not truly separate but coexist, or with the latter being an aspect or misperception of the former; often rendered as "spontaneous" or "spontaneity"; the sahaja state is the natural condition, that is, enlightenment or realization

Samadhi ("putting together") — the ecstatic or unitive state in which the meditator becomes one with the object of meditation; the eighth and final limb (anga) of Patanjali's eightfold path; there are many types of samadhi, the most significant distinction being between samprajnata (super-conscious) and asamprajnata (supra-conscious) ecstasy; only the latter leads to the dissolution of the karmic factors deep within the mind; beyond both types of ecstasy is enlightenment, which is also sometimes called sahaja-samâdhi or the condition of "natural" or "spontaneous" ecstasy, where there is perfect continuity of supra-conscious throughout waking, dreaming, and sleeping

Samatva ("evenness") — the mental condition of harmony, balance

Samkhya ("number") — one of the main philosophies of Yoga, which is concerned with the classification of the principles (tattva) of existence and their proper discernment in order to distinguish between Spirit (Purusha) and the various aspects of nature (prakriti); this influential system grew out of the ancient (pre-Buddhist) Samkhya Yoga tradition and was codified in the Samkhya-Karika of Îshvara Krishna (c. 350CE)

Samnyasa ("casting off") — the state of renunciation, which is the fourth and final stage of life (see ashram) and consisting primarily in an inner turning away from what is understood to be finite and secondarily in an external letting go of finite things; cf. vairâgya

Samnyasin ("he who has cast off") — a renunciate
Samprajnata-samadhi; see samâdhi
Samsara ("confluence") — the finite world of change, as opposed to the ultimate reality (brahman or nirvâna)
Samskara ("activator") — the subconscious impression left behind by each act of volition, which, in turn, leads to renewed psycho-mental activity; the countless samskaras hidden in the depth of the mind are ultimately eliminated only in asamprajnata-samâdhi (see samâdhi)
Samyama ("constraint") — the combined practice of concentration (dharana), meditation (dhyana), and ecstasy (samadhi) in regard to the same object
Sanjeevani — the yogic process of regeneration and lengthening of the life-span of the physical body, for specific spiritual work
Sapta Rishi — the Seven Primordial Sages, corresponding to the seven stars of the Great Bear
Sat ("truth") — the ultimate reality (Atman or Brahman)
Satguru ("one with gravity") — a Master who brings to light the Spiritual knowledge inherent in man; an enlightened aspect of the Divine Satsang ("fellowship of Truth") — the practice of frequenting the good company of saints, sages, Self-realized adepts, and their disciples; mentioned in the Yoga Vashisht as one of the four cornerstones to spiritual success.
Satya ("truth/truthfulness") — truth, a designation of the ultimate reality; also the practice of truthfulness, which is an aspect of moral discipline (yama)
Sevak — servant of humanity; a hamsasevak is one who has received the 1st level of initiation
Shakti ("power") — the kinetic aspect of the potential Shiva (God-realization), the power to transform and evolve aspirants to this enlightened state; see also kundalini shakti
Shaktipat ("descent of shakti") — one of the three blessings (shivapat, shaktipat, and pranapat) Sat-Gurunath bestows upon his disciples for their spiritual progress; the awakening of the dormant kundalini energy of a disciple.
Shambalpur (Shambala) where Siva-Goraksha-Babaji reigns as

Spiritual King until the world cycle is over; its higher center is in the aurora borealis of the Northern Lights

Shishya ("chela/disciple") — the initiated disciple of a Guru

Shiva ("the Benevolent One") — the Consciousness of the universe. The great destroyer of delusion and spiritual rejenerator of mankind. He is the Divine potential aspect of his own kinetic Shakti energy; also called Mahadeva (Great God)

Shivapat ("Shiva's grace") — the Sat-Guru, as Consciousness and The Presence, awares himself into the mind-disciple, transforming that mind into his own Consciousness to the degree of the disciple's receptivity to his Consciousness; cf. pranapat, shaktipat

Shiva-Sûtra ("Shiva's Aphorisms") — like the Yoga-Sûtra of Patanjali, a classical work on Yoga, as taught in the Shaivism of Kashmir; authored by Vasugupta (ninth century C.E.)

Shodhana ("cleansing/purification") — a fundamental aspect of all yogic paths; a category of purification practices in Hatha Yoga

Shraddhâ ("faith") — an essential disposition on the yogic path, which must be distinguished from mere belief

Shuddhi ("purification/purity") — the state of purity; a synonym of shodhana

Shvetdeep – ("White Island"); see Shambalpur

Siddha ("accomplished") — a perfected Master; an adept; the term mahasiddha or "great adept" should only be used for the Nine Immortal Naths

Siddhi ("accomplishment/perfection") — spiritual perfection, the attainment of flawless identity with the ultimate reality (atman or brahman); paranormal ability, of which the Yoga tradition knows many kinds

Stitha-pradnya (Sthita-prajna) – ("he who is steadied in wisdom"), the sage who is content abiding in the Self alone, who has expelled all desire and is neither dismayed by sorrowful events nor elated by joyous experiences

Sushumna-nadi ("very gracious channel") — the central prana current in or along which the serpent power (kundalini shakti) must ascend toward the psycho-energetic center (chakra) at the crown of the head in order to attain liberation (moksha)

Sutra ("thread") — an aphoristic statement; a work consisting of aphoristic statements, such as Patanjali's Yoga-Sûtras or Vasugupta's Shiva-Sûtra

Svadhyaya ("one's own going into") — study, an important aspect of the yogic path, listed among the practices of self-restraint (niyama) in Patanjali's eightfold Yoga; the recitation of mantras (see also japa)

Swaroop (svaroop) — embodiment of one's true Self; the essential nature of a thing

Swashan-Jwala — Breath of fire; a pranayama technique involving the forceful breathing through each nostril and the mouth

Swayambhoo — the "Great Unborn" (aja), Self-manifestation and personal aspect of Lord Shiva. The Cosmic Being Babaji- Gorakshanath will not incarnate from age to age, but is perpetually present until the world cycle (Mahakalpa) is over. He broods over humanity, his children, from eternity to eternity and is thus known as "the Great acrifice". His work is far beyond the comprehension of mortals

T

Tanmatra (tanu-matra "fine matter") — the subtle aspect of the material elements (bhuta) which may be seen in the form of light during yoni-mudra (also jyoti-mudra); the potentials of sound (shabda), form (rupa), touch (sparsha), taste (rasa), and smell (gandha)

Tantra ("Loom") — a classical Indian work containing Tantric teachings; the tradition of Tantrism, which focuses on the shakti aspect of spiritual life (originated in the early post-Christian era) and achieved its classical features around 1000CE; Tantrism has a "right-hand" (dakshina) or conservative and a "left-hand" (vâma) or unconventional branch, with the latter utilizing, among other things, sexual rituals

Tapas ("glow/heat") — austerity or endurance of extremes, an element of all yogic approaches, since they all involve renunciation and transcendence

Tapasvi (Tapasvin) — A practicioner of tapas, the endurance of extremes, austerity

Tattva ("thatness") — a fact or reality; a particular category of existence such as the ahamkara, buddhi, manas; the ultimate reality (see also Atman, Brahman)

Turiya ("fourth"), also called Cathurtha — the transcendental reality, which exceeds the three conventional states of consciousness, namely waking, sleeping, and dreaming

U

Unmani — no-mind state; a state of thoughtless awareness

Upanishad ("sitting near") — a classical Indian scripture representing the conclusion of the "revealed literature" of Sanatana Dharma (‚the Vedas), hence the designation Vedanta for the teachings of these sacred works; cf. Aranyaka, Brahmana, Veda

V

Vairagya ("dispassion") — the attitude of inner renunciation, the counterpole to abhyâsa

Vak also Vac ("speech") — Divine speech; the power of manifestation; there are four vak, vaikhari (loud sound), madhyama (murmuring sound), pashyanti (mental sound), para (meditative unheard sound); Vak is also a name of Sarasvati, Vak Sarasvati

Vasana ("trait") — the constenation of subliminal activators (samskara) deposited in the depth of the mind where they exert a binding effect

Vastu Gyan — the science of geomancy involving the proper directions for architecture: homes, temples, buildings, etc; attributed to Vishvakarma, the architect of the Gods. The Chinese took these ancient Indian records and translated them into the science Feng-Shui.

Vastuspati Shiva — the planet Sirius; the hunter (Vyad) who slays the deer (Mrugnakshatra, the constellation Orion). From this originated the science of Vastu Gyan "geomancy"

Veda ("knowledge") — the body of sacred wisdom found in the four Vedic hymnodes that form the source of Hinduism: Rig-Veda, Yajur- Veda, Sâma-Veda, and Atharva-Veda; also the collective name for these hymnodies; cf. Vedanta

Vedanta ("Veda's end") — the teachings forming the doctrinal conclusion of the revealed literature (shruti) of Sanatana Dharma; see also Upanishad; cf. Aranyaka, Brahmana, Veda

Videha-mukti ("disembodied liberation") — the state of liberation without a physical or subtle body; cf. jîvan-mukti

Vidya ("knowledge/wisdom") — a synonym of prajna

Vishnu ("pervader") — the preserver; worshipped by Vaishnavas and who has had nine incarnations, including Rama and Krsna, with the tenth incarnation (avatara) Kalki coming at the start of the Aquarian age

Viveka ("discernment") — the aspect of the yogic path involving discrimination between the Self and the not-self (Truth and falsehood); "Incernment" - coined by Yogiraj SatGurunath Siddhanth

Vritti ("whirl") — in Patanjali's yoga-darshana, specifically the five types of mental activity: valid cognition (pramana), misconception (viparyaya), imagination (vikalpa), sleep (nidra), and memory (smriti)

Vyasa ("Arranger") — name of several great sages, but specifically referring to Veda Vyasa, who arranged the Vedic hymns in their current form and who also is attributed with the compilation of the Puranas, the Mahabharata, and other works, including the commentary on the Yoga-Sutras of Patanjali, Yoga-Bhashya

Y

Yajna ("sacrifice") — ritual fire sacrifice involving the chanting of mantras and shlokas. Yoga also knows of an inner sacrifice of kindling the internal flame of kundalini.

Yajnavalkya — the most renowned sage of the early Upanishadic era

Yama ("discipline") — the first "limb" (anga) of Patanjali's eightfold path, comprising moral precepts that have universal validity (such as non-harming and truthfulness); also the name of the gatekeeper of the netherworld, Yama "the First Mortal".

Yantra ("device") — a geometric design representing the body of one's meditation deity, used for external and internal concentration and worship

Yoga ("union/discipline") — the practice of the union of the individual Soul (Jiva) with the Supreme Spirit (Shiva); the unitive discipline by which inner freedom is sought; spiritual practice, as practiced in Hinduism, Buddhism, and Jainism, and transcending all religons; the spiritual tradition originated in India

Yoga-darshana ("Yoga view/system") — Patanjali's Raja-Yoga

Yoga-Sutra ("Aphorisms of Yoga") — Patanjali's aphoristic compilation forming a source of Raja-Yoga

Yogi — a male practitioner of Yoga

Yogini — a female practitioner of Yoga

Yogiraj – "King of yogis;" a title of exaltation and praise granted to a spiritual Master

Yoni ("womb") — the perineum or female genitalia; also the source of the universe, the primordial deep; cf. linga

Yoni mudra – also known as jyoti mudra, and shan-mukhi-mudra; the blocking of one's ears, eyes, and nostrils with one's fingers where the inner sound, anahata-nada (omkar) is heard and the Soul and seen as a spot of light at the third eye

Yuga ("age/era") — a division of time; as expounded by Swami Sri Yukteswar, the four ages of ascending and descending arcs (12,000 years in length), forming one Mahayuga of 24,000 years.

More Books By
Yogiraj Gurunath Siddhanath

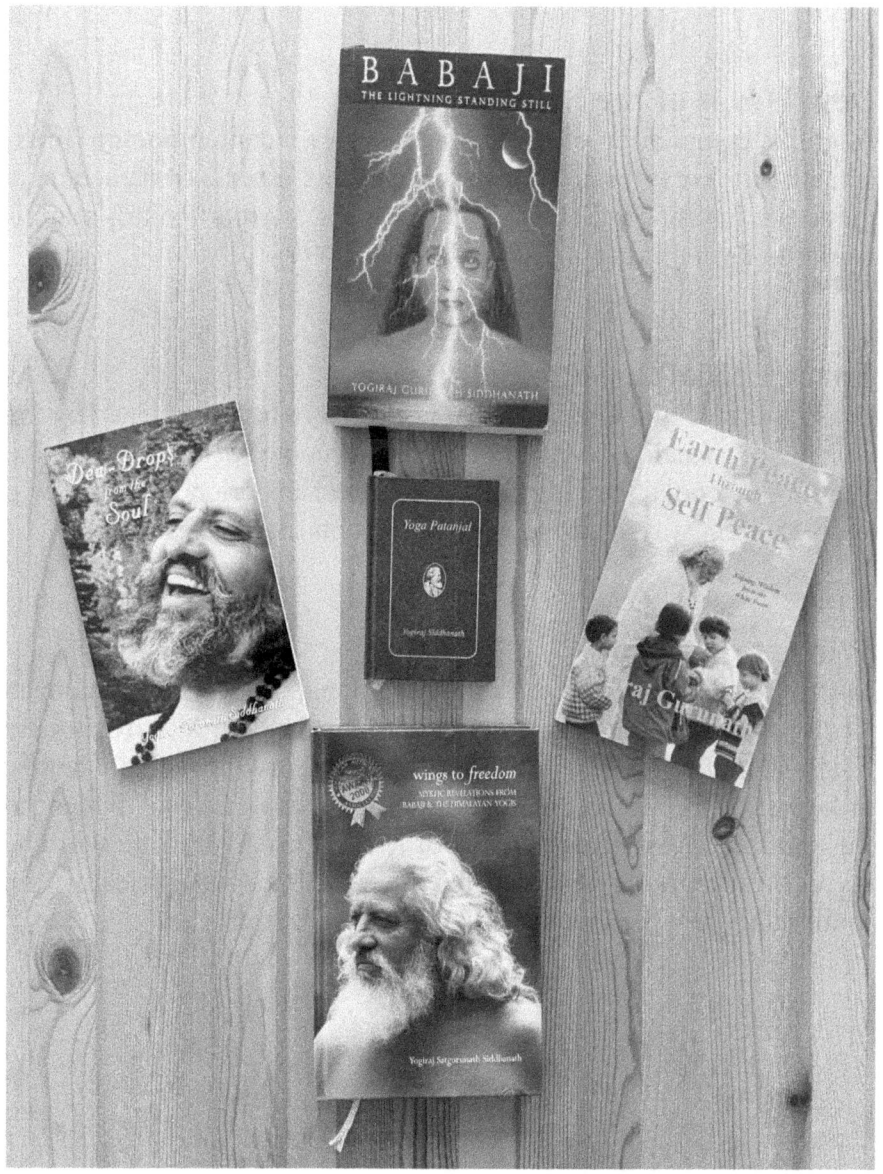

Books by Yogiraj Gurunath Siddhanath

Dew-Drops of the Soul
A unique compilation of poetical gems from a contemporary Himalayan Master, expressing the essence of his inner experience, as a guide and inpiration for all spiritual seekers. It is particularly illuminating to those practicing Kriya Yoga.

Earth Peace Through Self Peace
Grasp this splendid and unique opportunity to be enlightened by the wisdom of a Realized Master of Yoga. Gurunath speaks not from the learning of books, but from his own direct experience, in his own simple, direct way, clearing away all doubts and irrelevancies.

Wings to Freedom
Mystic revelations from the immortal Babaji and other Himalayan Yogis, as experienced by a perfected Master, Yogiraj SatGurunath Siddhanath. Follow his footsteps and experience through his words, as he walks his talk, in the jungles, temples, ashrams and hidden [to the uninitiated] spiritual vortices of India. Enrich your life with the secret oral traditions revealed for the first time - mysteries of life, immortality and the attainment of Self-Realization.

Babaji The Lightning Standing Still
This is the most in depth exposition of the the greatest enigmatic mystery of spiritual myth, legend and history, called Babaji in recent times and Gorakshanath in the ancient times. Yogiraj calls Him,'the Non-Being Essentiality.'

Shiva-Goraksha-Babaji is the ever appearing disappearing star of salvation to all humans and celestials alike. He is the lightning standing still who transforms himself into the star each time a soul is enlightened.

Yogiraj was personally transformed and enlightened by Babaji and is able to reveal the many hidden dimensions of this glorious Being.

Yoga Patanjal
For thousands of years, the yoga sutras attributed to Rishi Patanjali has been the premier text for all those who aspired to understand the spiritual evolution of consciousness towards Self-Realization. Yogiraj, from his own experience, has offered an illuminating commentary that stands unique in the annals of yogic tradition wherein he has been able to reveal hidden aspects of the original terse text.